The Autistic Spectrum
Parents' Daily Helper

A Workbook for
You and Your Child

Philip Abrams
Leslie Henriques, M.P.H.

FOREWORD BY
LORNA WING, M.D.

Ulysses Press
Berkeley, California

Published by: Ulysses Press
                P.O. Box 3440
                Berkeley, CA 94703
                www.ulyssespress.com

Library of Congress Control Number: 2003109419
ISBN: 1-56975-386-5

Printed in Canada by Transcontinental Printing

10 9 8 7 6 5 4 3 2 1

Editorial and production staff: Ashley Chase, Claire Chun, Lily Chou
Cover design: Sarah Levin
Interior design: Leslie Henriques
Cover Photograph: Michelle and Philip Abrams
Illustrations: Some images © 2004 from Hemera.com; some images © 2004 from www.clipart.com

Distributed in the United States by Publishers Group West and in Canada by Raincoast Books

The authors have made every effort to trace copyright owners. Where they have failed, they offer their apologies and undertake to make proper acknowledgment where possible in reprints.

This book has been written and published strictly for informational purposes, and in no way should it be used as a substitute for consultation with professional therapists. All facts in this book came from scientific publications, personal interviews, published trade books, self-published materials by experts, magazine articles, and the personal-practice experiences of the authorities quoted or sources cited. The authors and publisher are providing you with information in this work so that you can have the knowledge and can choose, at your own risk, to act on that knowledge.

To Elijah,
for opening our eyes and hearts.

Acknowledgments

First, I want to recognize the staff at Ulysses Press for their support during the endless process of putting this book together. Claire, the midwife of this book, put things together, as always. Sarah Levin added her talents with the cover. A special nod to editor Ashley Chase for diplomatically handling this assignment moments after she walked through the office door. She took our labor of love and crafted it into a practical tool for parents and children.

Lorna Wing graciously encouraged us while we were writing this book. It was her book, *The Autistic Spectrum,* that gave us the idea to create a workbook for parents. Her assistance and kindness through the years has been a source of inspiration.

Gaga, Ken, Nancy as well as my close friends and family, thank you for being there. Vicki Van Hanson needs to be singled out for her years of friendship.

Aloha Ray, Alice, Keith, my precious family, for sustaining me with take-out meals, words of wisdom, laughter and love. *Mahalo nui loa.* I could not have done this without you.

This book would not be a reality if it were not for my co-author and remarkable brother, Phil. You and Michelle are the most patient parents I have known. How lucky VeraRose and Elijah are to have you to start them on their journey through life. It's been an honor working with you.

—L.H.

Thanks to Ulysses Press for creating the opportunity to share some of my experiences and to convey my son's unique awareness and perspective of life.

Much gratitude to all who have helped us on this remarkable journey and all the love and learning that you have bestowed on us and Elijah—especially the folks at Cheerful Helpers who have been an invaluable support for our whole family.

An enormous thanks to our friends and to our extended family without whose love and support we would not be able to get through each day—most importantly, Gaga, Maja and Paja. Thanks to all our siblings for their love and grace, especially my dear sister Leslie for working so laboriously to make this book a reality.

My greatest love and thanks goes to my little family—Michelle, my darling wife, VeraRose, my peanut, and, of course, Elijah A.

—P.A.

Table of Contents

PART THREE: Tear-outs

Foreword

It gives me much pleasure to write the preface for this workbook. A professional in the field of autistic spectrum disorders, I am also a parent. My grown-up daughter has typical Kanner's autism. When she was a small child, little was known about autism, and there was virtually nowhere for parents to find helpful advice. In fact, it was the era when psychoanalytical theories of autism predominated, and blaming the parents was in fashion.

How things have changed since those days. In place of armchair theorizing, scientists have carried out objective research on autism and established that it is a developmental disorder due to biological causes. Pioneering parents refused to accept the idea that they had caused their child's autism. They joined together in voluntary associations and passed on to each other useful methods for helping their children, methods learned from their own experiences.

The authors of this workbook follow in that tradition. Phil Abrams is the parent of Elijah, who has autism. As well as working with his own son, Phil has trained to work with other children who have this developmental disorder. Leslie Henriques is Phil's sister and, as Elijah's aunt, is much involved with him. This workbook is the very positive outcome of these experiences.

The authors have taken on board three important facts about children with any type of autistic spectrum disorder. First, such children have a desperate need for life to follow a predictable, set routine. Second, they are distressed by anything new and unexpected. New experiences must be introduced gradually through links with familiar things. Third, they have severe problems in understanding concepts that are at all complicated, especially if presented in spoken words. They find it much easier to cope with concrete pictures or, if they can read, written words.

The workbook is designed to take these basic issues into account, with simple pictures and texts that illustrate each daily task or experience in small concrete steps. One of the book's strengths is that the authors are not wedded to any single educational method—they go for what works in practice. They recognize that each child with autism is a unique person with her own special needs, as well as special skills and interests.

One particularly useful feature are the sample pictures and labels, which the authors suggest replacing with specific images and content familiar to the child. This is especially appropriate for the second part of the book, which gives suggestions for helping each child build up a workbook of his own, providing a visual record of everyday experiences. I was very happy to see that the authors include fun and games for the children as well as the serious tasks of everyday life. So much of life is distressing for children with autistic spectrum disorders; it is wonderful to be able to make them laugh and enjoy some activities.

The workbook is aimed at more able children. Because the autistic spectrum includes children with such a wide range of abilities and needs, it is appropriate for a practical book of this kind to be aimed at a specific subgroup. It would be most welcome if the publication of this book were to lead to workbooks as good as this one becoming available for other subgroups.

Lorna Wing, M.D.
Psychiatric Consultant,
National Autistic Society (U.K.)

Preface

My mother was the first to say something. I certainly didn't think the conversation she started was going to pertain to my *perfect* son's development. She kicked it off by asking me if I thought there might be a problem with Eli's hearing. I asked why and she said, "Because he never turns to look at me when I call his name."

"He's just busy," I responded, adding, "Besides, he doesn't hang out with you that often, so he doesn't really know you. Why would he respond to you?" I didn't mean to slight her, but I didn't know what else to say. She wanted to pay for a hearing test and then offered to pay for some *other* tests. She handed me a huge stack of papers my brother had printed off the internet about children with PDD, Pervasive Developmental Disorder—a category of developmental disorders that includes the autistic spectrum.

That evening my wife and I jokingly made up our own acronyms for PDD: "Perfectly Delightful and Delicious," etc. We were in denial. How were we to know the way a toddler is supposed to act? Eli was our first child, and we just thought he was very focused, a quality that seemed to bode well for his future success. He smiled and laughed— but he didn't talk. Maybe he was simply a late talker, we told ourselves. My brother even offered up a book about late talkers and how exceptional they were. Yes, my son is exceptional, but not because he was a late talker. Instead, it's because he has special needs.

Eli was good at zoning out for long stretches of time. It was very difficult to engage him in an activity that was not to his liking, or even to understand what he wanted at any given moment. Sometimes we would pick up every object on the table and offer each one to him in turn, hoping at last to find the one he was grunting for.

It wasn't until a horrendous experience at a day camp—Eli spent most of the time screaming in the doorway—that we finally took the plunge and had him tested by a developmental pediatrician. The results were hard to swallow: he was diagnosed with Autistic Spectrum Disorder. We were told we had to act fast if we were going to break into his world, which was slowly but surely shutting our world out.

And so our journey began. We moved slowly at first, very slowly. We had no idea where to get help, and the first assistance was less than satisfactory. We didn't really understand our son's condition for a long time. It seemed that every time we turned around there was some revolutionary new treatment or explanation for autism. Now we understand that nobody really knows the answer to the question "What is autism?" Some methods work for one child, others work for another.

What worked for Eli was spending time around people with lots of personality. That "high affect" manner was key to getting him engaged. Fortunately, my wife and I both have personalities that work well with our son's needs. I am an actor, so reaching out and engaging people comes naturally. Whenever someone new came into our lives to work with Eli, our first question was: "Is his personality *big* enough?" It wasn't long before Eli's first "big personality" behaviorist came along. Misten had a gift and helped Eli to emerge partially from the world that is the size of his body—she connected with him and he with her.

Toward the end of her stint with us, Misten mentioned that the workload at her agency was too large, with many kids on the waiting list and not enough people to work with them. The agency needed help. I thought about it for a couple of weeks and then out of the blue asked, "How about me?" She smiled and responded, "I have been waiting for you to ask. You are very good with Eli, and I think you would be great with other kids. You are a natural."

That's how I found my new vocation as a behaviorist and play therapist. I had lots of hands-on experience with my own son. I trained under Misten and took some ABA (Applied Behavior Analysis) workshops. I then started working with a boy one year younger than Eli who had many of the same behaviors as my son. Five years later I still work with that boy, and it has been a rewarding experience to see his growth and development. I have several other clients now, and even though I sometimes feel as if I don't know what

I am doing—because this work is often more art than science—I still marvel at the progress of these children. Now I am a behaviorist, a play therapist, an actor and a father still learning how to unlock my own son's mysteries.

Even though I can't imagine exactly what it is like, I know that my son experiences the world very differently than I do. Certainly, everyone has an individual perspective on the world—but as I continue to research neurological variations that present challenges, I realize that some people go through life with a very marked difference in awareness, perception and sensitivity. Jim Sinclair is a disability rights activist and writer who has autism. This is what he has to say about the autistic perspective:

> Autism isn't something a person has, or a "shell" that a person is trapped inside. There's no normal child hidden behind the autism. Autism is a way of being. It is pervasive; it colors every experience, every sensation, perception, thought, emotion and encounter, every aspect of existence. It is not possible to separate the autism from the person—and if it were possible, the person you'd have left would not be the same person you started with.

My son's unique perspective has brought the world into sharper focus for me. Eli's experience of the world is immediate. He doesn't engage the future the way we do; he is too encumbered by the present. So when his joy is great, it is really great—and when his pain (emotional or psychological) is great, it is *really great*. I hope I can embrace the present the way Eli does, experiencing the moment and cherishing it with grace. This is the gift, the blessing and the trial that life has handed to me. Even though it can feel like a weight at times, I would never trade it for the world.

The seminal moment in our lives occurred recently when Elijah, in his haltingly expressive voice, chimed out, "I'm happy to be in the world." We were elated. Our hope with this book is to assist you on your journey so that one day your whole family can enthusiastically say, "We're happy to be in the world." Although he has a long way to go in understanding many of the concepts we take for granted—time, expression of feelings, safety issues, to name a few—Eli is on the road moving forward.

Philip Abrams
Leslie Henriques

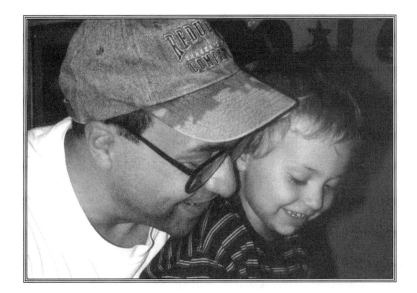

Author Philip Abrams with his son, Elijah

How to Use This Book

If you are reading this book, you have probably already begun your journey as a parent or caregiver of a child with autism. Our journey into the world of autism began when Elijah was diagnosed on the autistic spectrum at 22 months of age. Nobody can be prepared for such a journey. What do you pack? Our family's bags were empty, but even after five years they are being crammed with new information daily.

This book is designed to assist those who have a basic understanding of autism and who could benefit from some straightforward strategies to help their child navigate everyday life. If you are looking for a comprehensive book about autism, you might read Dr. Lorna Wing's *The Autistic Spectrum*. (See Resources on page 79 for more information on autism.)

As you are probably aware, the autistic spectrum encompasses a remarkably wide range of children. This book is geared toward parents of "high-functioning" children. If your child's disabilities are more severe, you may find that other methods are better suited to your needs.

Most of my experience with autism has come from life with my son. For the past five years I have also worked with other children on the autistic spectrum, and I am working toward a master's degree in Special Education. Still, unlike many other professionals, my life experience has been my greatest teacher. So I come to you as a parent first and foremost, and an educator second.

This book is not meant to stay neat and clean on the shelf. This is a hands-on book that should be taken apart and used. The pages in

WHAT IS THE AUTISTIC SPECTRUM?

The autistic spectrum includes a wide range of disabilities, including Kanner's autism, Asperger's syndrome and PDD (Pervasive Developmental Disorder). Children on the autistic spectrum show impairment in social interaction, communication and development of symbolic or imaginative play.

Part Two and Part Three are perforated for easy removal. These pages can also be photocopied and used multiple times. Once removed, pages can be three-hole punched and placed in a binder. You may want to laminate pages that you use over and over, such as the clock face, reinforcement tokens and choice cards.

The following items will help you get the most out of this book:
- Three-ring binders (one for you and one for your child)
- Scissors
- Glue (stick)
- Three-hole punch
- Zipper pouch to fit inside binder
- Camera
- Laminating machine (available for use at most copy shops), or you can use plastic sheet protectors

If you have been on the journey for any length of time, you probably already have a binder with your child's important papers from doctors, a developmental pediatrician, speech pathologist, occupational therapist and others. You can use that binder to include copies of the letters on pages 49 and 50.

Your child will benefit from having her own binder to keep her daily schedules protected. She can also keep some of the matching game pieces in a three-hole zip pouch inserted in the binder. Along with your child, discover which of the tear-out sheets are most helpful and keep those in the binder as well.

This book does not outline a specific method of treatment per se. Instead, we suggest a combination of relationship-based theory and behavioral techniques, along with a healthy dose of humor. This eclectic approach has been used in our family with great success. Still, it is important to remember that all children with autism are individuals. Children's manifestations of behavior might be somewhat similar, but they are all unique people who respond in different ways to different situations and different stimuli. No one knows your child better than you, so your task will be to discover what works best for your child. Alas, as we can attest, everyone must go through a process of trial and error to discover what is most effective. Even then, the most effective methods will change as weaknesses become strengths and new challenges are presented. This never-ending journey will take you deep into new territories of the heart.

A Note about Language

The English language does not make it easy to be gender-neutral. In order to include all children, male and female, we have alternated use of the pronouns *he* and *she*.

PART ONE

✣

Your Workbook

1

BREAKING THROUGH

Your first and most important challenge as the parent of a child on the autistic spectrum is reaching into your child's world and establishing communication. We've found that one of the most effective ways to "break through" is to use humor and play.

And why not? Laughter is one of the most powerful social forces in the human psychology. Laughter crosses all language and cultural barriers, so it makes sense that humor can help cross over the boundaries inherent to the child with autism. If you watch children with autism engaged in tickle-play, many respond with giggles and joy, as typical children do.

We have written the following exercises, games and pages in a spirit of humor and play. We hope you and your child will not only learn from them, but enjoy yourselves as well.

What Is Funny?

What makes your child laugh? What is your child's favorite toy? How can you use that toy in a humorous way so that you can break through the barrier and communicate? At first it might be difficult to figure out which styles of humor work best with your child. Keep searching, and you will discover some useful tricks. Still, no joke works forever, no matter how funny. Once the novelty wears off, your creativity must kick in. It's all about exploring new ways to bridge that gap.

Steps to laughter:

1) Observe your child and discover what his favorite toy is.

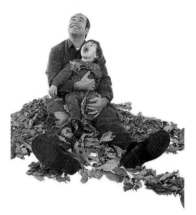

2) Get down on the floor with your child and use your hands playfully to "interrupt" his activity. I find that the use of funny sounds is one of the best ways to make a child laugh. Funny sounds include beeps, buzzes and the infamous passing wind noises.

3) Use his favorite toy in a way that is unexpected. (See The Incongruity Theory below.) Hide the toy and play peek-a-boo with it. Make-believe that *it* is creating the funny sounds that you are now using to great effect.

Interrupting activity and presenting playful obstacles are basic methods in floortime intervention. (See page 3.)

THE INCONGRUITY THEORY

One of the most common forms of humor is the use of surprise or incongruity. The incongruity theory states that humor arises when when the familiar and logical (*okay things*) are replaced by the unexpected (*not okay things*). When we expect one outcome and another happens, we experience two sets of incompatible thoughts and emotions (*okay and not okay*) simultaneously. This incongruity is viewed as humorous.

Connecting

One of your most important goals—perhaps *the* most important—should be to develop the relationship between your child's inner self and the outside world. Children on the autistic spectrum *are* very in touch with the emotional life that swirls around them, even though they might not show it in ways that are easy for us to recognize. Their behavior often mirrors their environment and the thoughts and feelings of the people who are most important in their lives.

This mirroring is the reason why it is so important for everyone who is providing services and support to your child to communicate clearly, honestly and thoughtfully. If you and the other members of your child's support system model effective communication, you will help your child learn to interact with the world.

FLOORTIME

Child psychiatrist Stanley Greenspan has created what he calls D.I.R.—a developmental, individual-difference, relationship-based approach to intervention, also known as "floortime." Here's a brief breakdown.

OBSERVATION: Listen to your child's tone of voice and watch her facial expressions and posture to figure out how to approach her.

OPEN CIRCLES OF COMMUNICATION: Acknowledge your child's emotional tone and then build on what she's doing at the moment.

FOLLOW THE CHILD'S LEAD: Be a play partner with your child. Narrate her play and let her be the leader.

EXTEND AND EXPAND PLAY: Ask a question and make a "twist" in the play so you have created an opportunity for her to react.

CHILD CLOSES THE CIRCLE OF COMMUNICATION: When she responds she has closed the circle. Remember, one circle opens you up to more circles of building communication; keep the circles opening and closing.

Hints on Ways to Establish Communication with Your Child

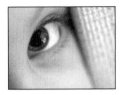 ☺ Literally see eye-to-eye with him. That often means squatting, sitting or even stretching out on the floor to make eye contact.

☺ Get close to your child: Determine what distance is physically acceptable for her. (Some kids like in-your-face closeness; others need about a foot of distance to feel relaxed.)

☺ Make eye contact whenever you are trying to communicate. You may need to move into your child's field of vision, or you may even need to turn his head.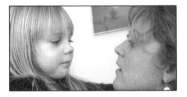

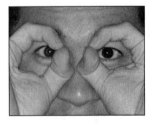 ☺ Play. Play. Play. Be rollicking, witty and fun! Your face and body should be as animated as possible. Children (all children) respond better to playfulness and the use of humor than to anything else.

☺ Use visual cues whenever possible. If your child responds better to auditory cues, use music and songs to communicate.

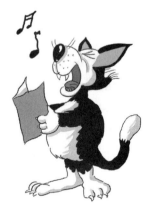

☺ Use your body language to communicate. I'm an actor, so I know how important body language is in communicating to an audience. Your child is your audience. You're on stage! She can relate better if you speak with your face and body as well as with words. Aim for that Oscar.

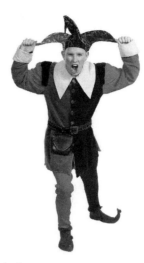

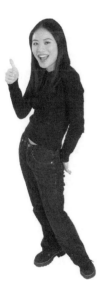

☺ Use gestures. Gesturing reinforces your communication. For example, when your child does something correctly give him a thumbs up while nodding and saying "Yes, good job." Or when you want him to stop what he is doing, put your hand out gesturing a halt, shake your head no and say, "Terry, look at me. You must stop now."

"Laughter is the shortest distance between two people."

—VICTOR BORGE

Transitions and Handling the Unexpected

As you know, children with autism do not easily tolerate transitions—moving from one activity to another. Much of the anxiety that surrounds these moments might have to do with the fear of the unknown. Because your child might not know what is coming next and cannot conceptualize time (see page 13), her anxiety increases
exponentially: "What is going to happen? When is it going to happen? When will it stop?" These might be a few of the questions that are racing around inside her brain. Her inability to voice these thoughts probably only adds to the fear that is mounting inside, and that fear often leads to inappropriate behavior.

You can use a variety of strategies to make transitions easier.

▲ Creating schedules that help your child understand time (see page 15)

▲ Using visual aids to show him what to expect (see page 28)

▲ Incorporating relaxation techniques (such as deep breathing)

▲ Exposing your child to new situations gradually (desensitizing)

▲ Applying deep pressure (a full-body squeeze can sometimes be extremely helpful in reorganizing your child's experience)

▲ Providing a "safe spot" (a place where your child can escape if a transition is too stressful)

Making Choices

When your child makes a choice, he interacts with the world. Even a simple choice involves a give-and-take with the child's environment. The act of making his own choice gives your child a feeling of autonomy. If you give your child many opportunities to make choices, you will help him develop independence and self-assurance.

You don't have to offer a large number of alternatives—that can sometimes be overwhelming. If you narrow down the choice to two or three options, it will be easier for your child to understand what selections are available.

On the next page are Choice Cards that you and your child can use to choose an activity for a period of free time. You can limit the choices by removing or covering up any choice cards you do not want to make available. The pictures of activities can be presented on a single sheet of paper or cut out and placed in a stack. You can even turn the choosing of an activity into a game by placing the cards face down on the table, letting your child turn cards over one by one to hunt for the preferred activity. (See Part Three for cutouts of choice cards.)

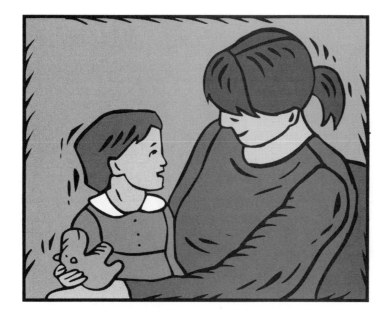

CHOICE CARDS

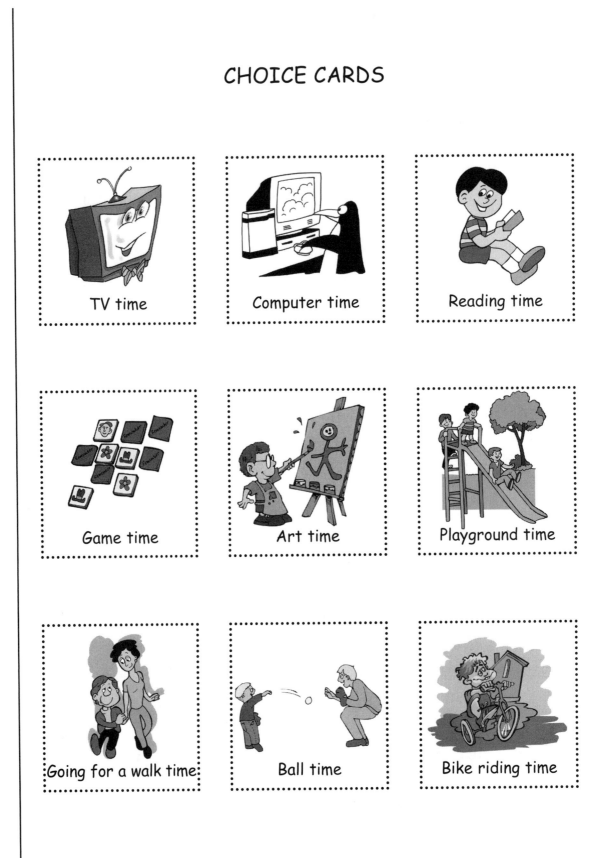

Prompting Your Child to Make Choices

These everyday activities will help build self-esteem and encourage creative play.

◘ While riding in the car, have your child choose a song to sing or a story to listen to on tape.

◘ When it's time to dress, give your child choices about what to wear. Put out two outfits that are appropriate for the day and ask your child to choose the ones she wants to put on.

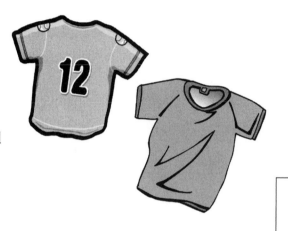

◘ Give your child a choice about what to take off first when undressing. This is a good time to talk about how you must take off the things on the outside first.

◘ When preparing a snack, give your child a choice between two or three different kinds of food.

◘ At bathtime, offer a choice of toys to play with in the tub. You can also offer different colors of towels, helping her to learn her colors and giving her options at the same time.

Visual aids will help your child a great deal when it's time to make a choice.

Reading Faces

One of the disabilities associated with autism is often called "mindblindness." This is an inability to read emotions and feelings on other people's faces, and it can present difficulties in interpersonal relationships. In helping to create relationships, a sense of empathy is important. Empathy can only be achieved if your child knows what emotions or feelings another person is experiencing.

Distinguishing basic facial expressions is a useful skill. You will find a matching game on the next page designed to help your child "read" faces. Cover the words up and ask your child to point to the faces that express the various emotions. As always, humor and an animated, lively manner will make the game more effective. (Other face-reading games can be found in Part Two.)

One game you can play without cards or props is to act out emotions yourself. Exaggerate the emotions in a humorous way and encourage your child to imitate your actions.

A small hand-held mirror can be an effective teaching tool. Your child can "wear" an emotion and look in the mirror to see what that looks like on his own face. The mirror is also invaluable when your child is having a real emotional experience. You can help him see his emotional expression; this will help him to communicate what he feels.

Expressing feelings verbally is often a daunting task for a child on the autistic spectrum. These are just some ways of helping them to access visually what they might be experiencing internally. My *typical* three year-old is always looking in the mirror when she is "upset" to test out what it looks and feels like.

The use of play in the treatment of children with autism has been very effective in developing a relationship with the *world*.

MATCHING FACES

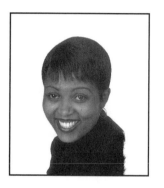

happy

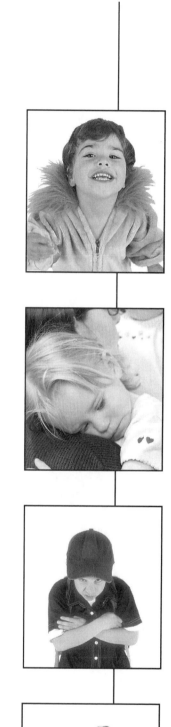

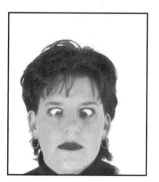

tired

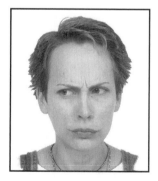

mad

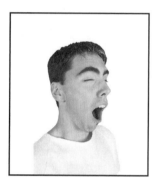

silly

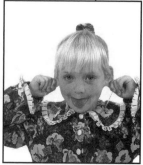

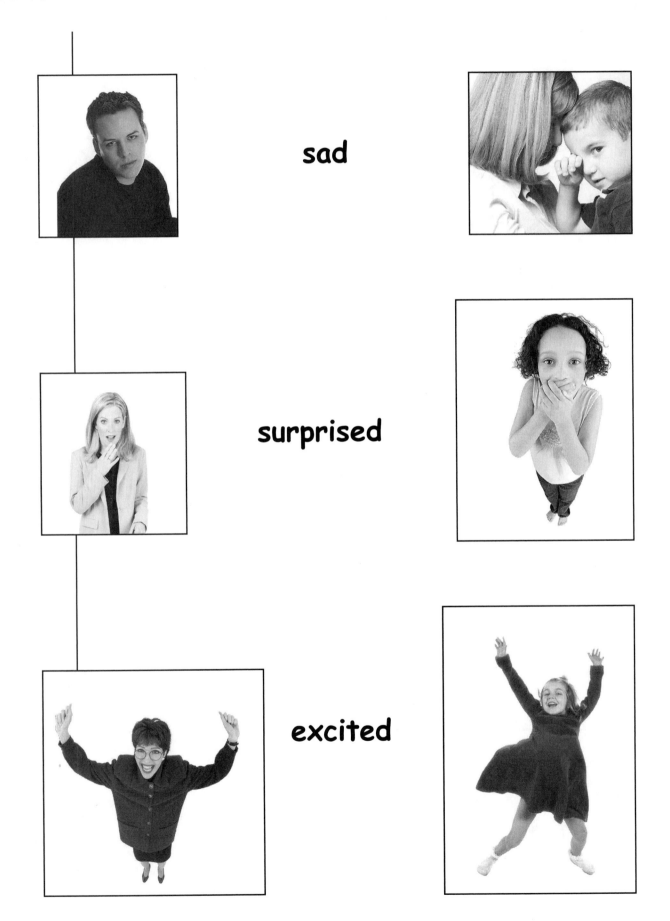

sad

surprised

excited

2

DEVELOPING A SENSE OF TIME AND PLACE

Unlike typical children, children on the autistic spectrum do not have an innate sense of time. They have difficulty conceiving the passage of time. In addition, there is a fundamental inability to make sense of past and present experiences. Imagine being in a sensory deprivation tank; you've lost the ability to distinguish where your body begins and ends and which way is up. The concept of time is something like that for a child on the autistic spectrum. He often isn't able to distinguish between past, present and future. Because he cannot comprehend *when*, your child might experience great anxiety when faced with not knowing *what* is going to happen next.

This is not to say that children on the spectrum are unable to tell you what time it is if they look at a clock. (Some are quite capable of learning to read a clock and may even have a higher comprehension of numbers than their typical peers.) The difficulty lies in recognizing the passage of time and linking it to ongoing activities. Careful planning can provide your child with the necessary tools to navigate his day, while maintaining an emotional equilibrium.

Life is complicated these days, for everyone. If you stop for a minute to think of all the tasks you do in a day—from preparing meals to visiting doctors and therapists to picking up children from various activities to getting children into bed and asleep (whew)—it can be pretty daunting. Many of us use lists to keep track of what we need to do. Lists help us manage our time and make sense of our busy lives. In the same way, lists (either visual or written) will help your child keep track of her day.

So often the sense of anxiety that a child with autism experiences stems from the unknown. Giving her something tangible to hold onto is an effective way to alleviate that anxiety. That is one of the ultimate goals of creating a Daily Binder, along with helping your child to develop a sense of time and place.

There are many things that can be kept in the binder:

• Daily Schedule

• Pictures

• "All About Me" pages

• Money sheets (for review in community settings)

Help your child to chose what is important for *his* binder.

Creating a Daily Binder for your child provides the added benefit of making *you* more organized. The pages that follow describe organizational strategies that have worked for us:

• Daily Schedules

• Mini-schedules

• Calendars

• Visual Cue Box

• Fridge Central

CHANGE IN ROUTINE

Your child's days are filled with changing situations, each with the possibility of causing her stress. One way to alleviate the stress of not knowing what is going to happen next is to create schedules. But as you are well aware, things happen, and schedules have to be adapted. It is important for your child to learn to incorporate change into her life.

One way to help her adjust to change is to prepare her for it. Create visual cues to alert her. For instance, you can use an icon such as ☞ or a Post-it note on her daily schedule to indicate "We're doing something different today." The note could be followed by a ☺ to suggest that change is okay.

Daily Schedules

In this section we provide examples of schedules, both visual and written. By creating schedules you can show your child what he will be doing during the day. This creates a sense of well-being and will help all of you.

Go over your child's schedule with him at the beginning of the day. This will make him more comfortable and less confused, and he can refer to his schedule any time he feels unsure of what is happening.

The first sample schedule is designed for a child who needs visual cues. If your child needs visual cues, create a book of schedules for her. Cut out the pictures in this book, or search through magazines with your child. Of course, taking photos of the places and people

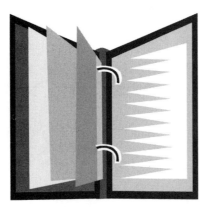

Changes to your daily routines need to be planned ahead of time and, if possible, introduced slowly, with ample preparation.

who are in your child's life is the most effective method. Then paste the images onto a sheet of paper in your own Daily Binder.

If your child is able to read, base your schedule on the second sample in this book. Have him keep the schedule in a pocket with him so that he can cross off the things that have occurred. Feel free to mix and match elements from the examples, depending on your child's level of understanding.

SAMPLE DAILY SCHEDULE 1

For cutouts of the timetable images, see pages 95–101.

Get up in the morning.

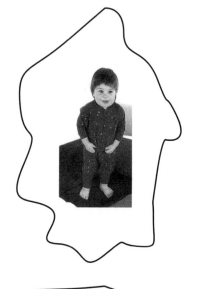

Use the toilet.

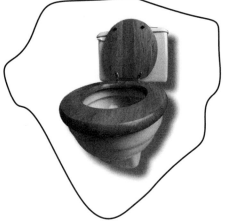

Eat breakfast.

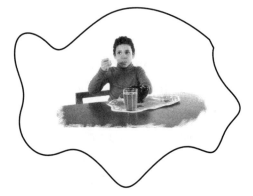

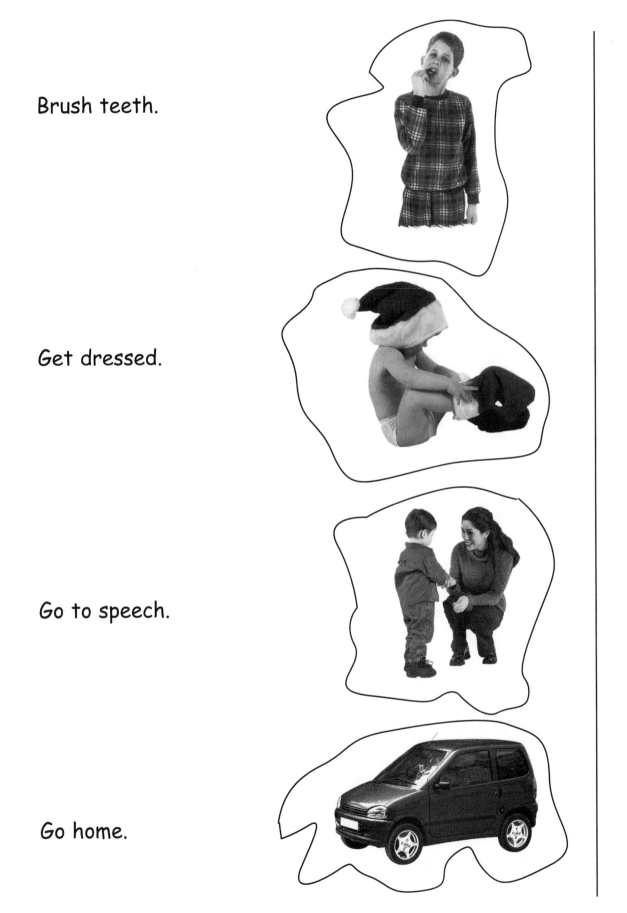

Brush teeth.

Get dressed.

Go to speech.

Go home.

Eat lunch.

Sometimes unexpected events occur. Try to come up with a method (visual, written or body language) to let your child know what is going to happen next in these situations.

Play with mom.

Read a book.

Have a snack.

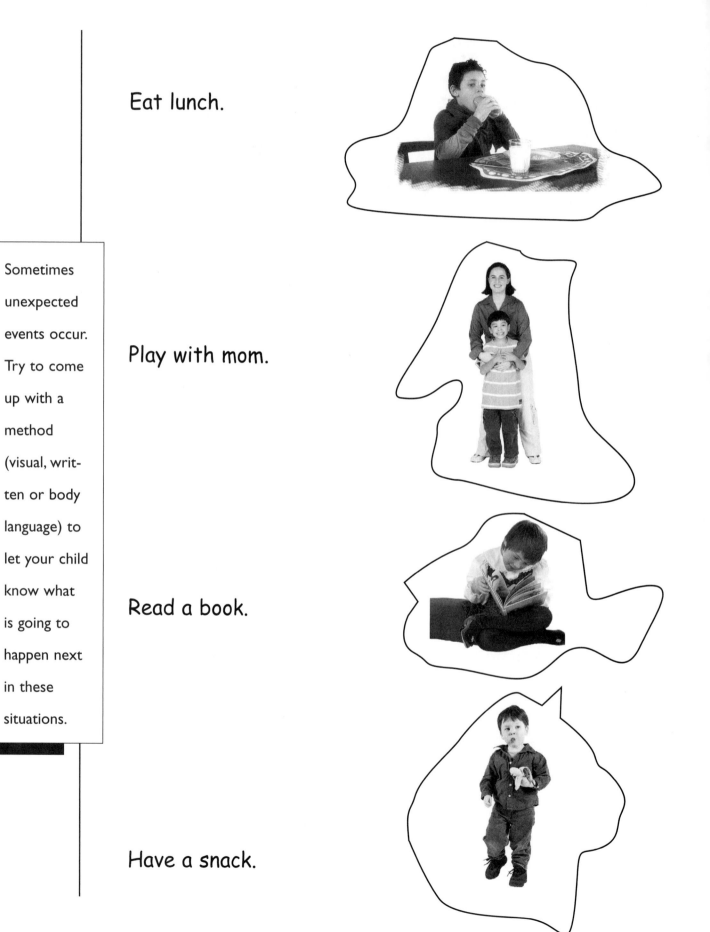

Mom comes home
with my sister.

Play with computer.

Eat dinner.

Get undressed.

Take a bath.

Regular exercise during the day may help your child sleep better at night.

Pajama time.

Watch videos.

Rock in a chair.

Go to bed.

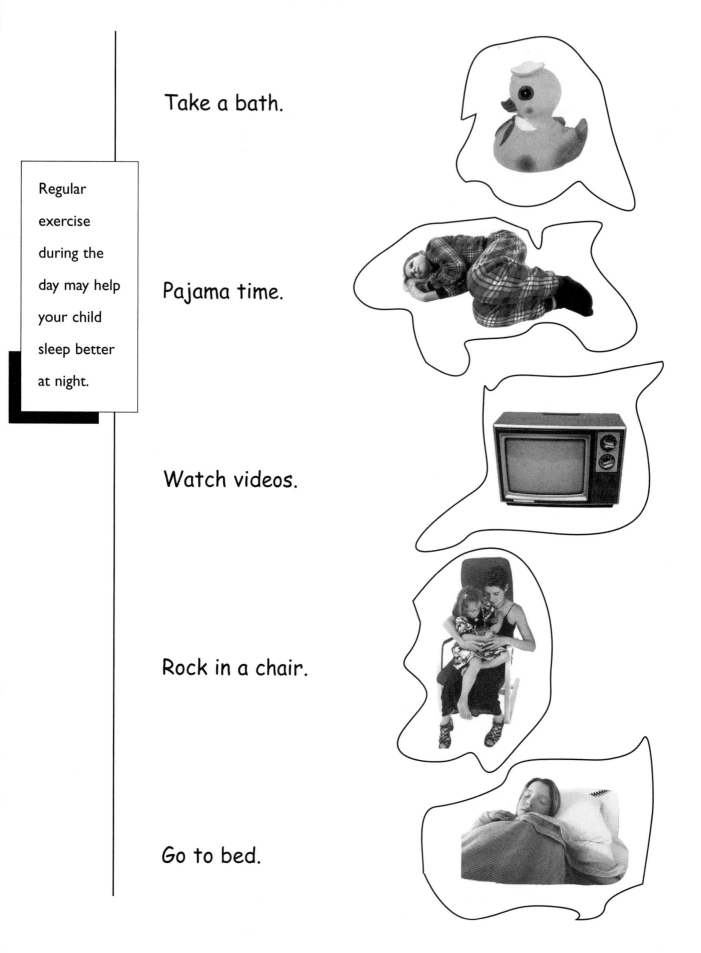

SAMPLE DAILY SCHEDULE 2

Here is an example of my son's schedule. It is geared for the child who can read. Most of the items are things he will do, but note that number six ("Mom comes home") instead lists an event that is important to him. Have your child read the list and cross out each item after it has occurred.

MY SCHEDULE

1. Watch PBS kids

2. Go to Stan's Donuts

3. Go to school

4. Come home & play

5. Lunch

6. Mom comes home

7. Swim at Maja's house

8. Dinner

9. Playtime

10. Bedtime

Mini-schedules

Mini-schedules can be used to help your child make the transition from one activity to another while making sure she has the information she needs to feel comfortable. They can also be used to teach your child the order of a skill, such as brushing teeth.

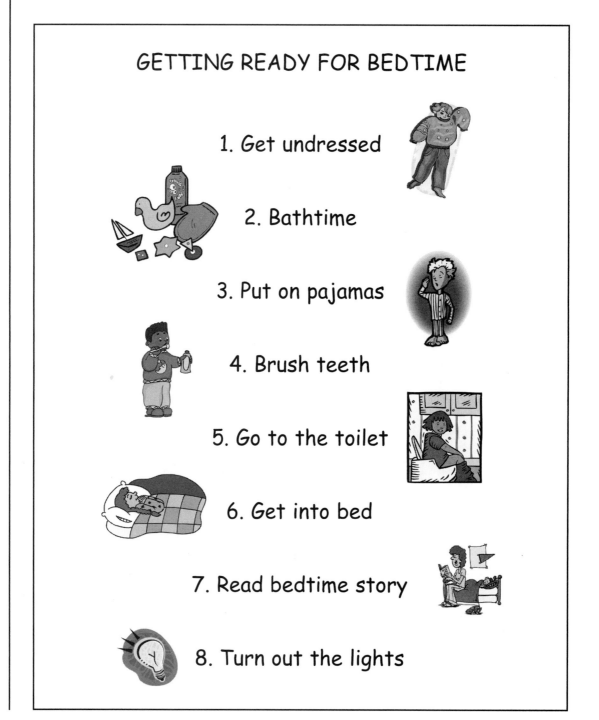

GETTING READY FOR BEDTIME

1. Get undressed

2. Bathtime

3. Put on pajamas

4. Brush teeth

5. Go to the toilet

6. Get into bed

7. Read bedtime story

8. Turn out the lights

SAMPLE: GETTING READY FOR BED VISUAL SCHEDULE

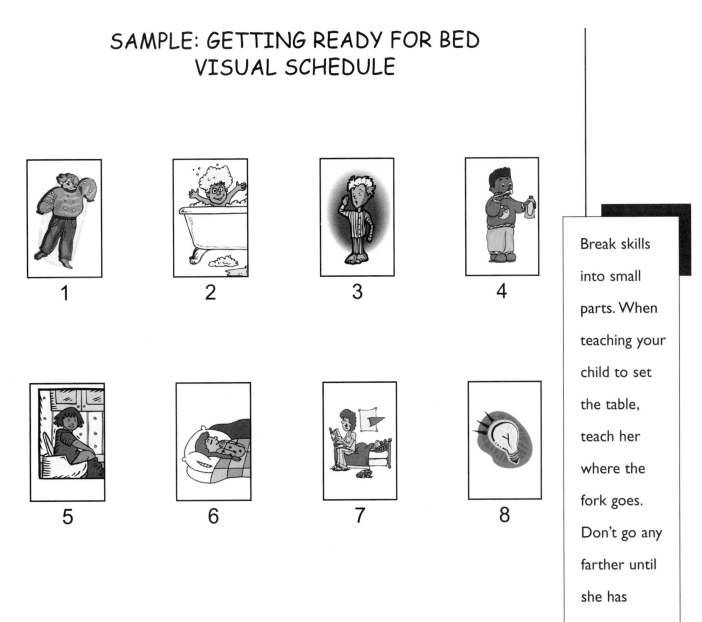

Break skills into small parts. When teaching your child to set the table, teach her where the fork goes. Don't go any farther until she has mastered that task.

Calendars

Calendars help your child visualize the concept of time passing. They alleviate anxiety because they show your child *what* will happen and *when* to expect it.

Create (or adapt) a monthly calendar for your child, marking important events with images or words. You will find a sample calendar on page 26. Coordinate the information on your child's daily schedules with the information on the calendar. This increases the scope of your child's perception of time and helps your child anticipate future activities. You can use a calendar to indicate a special event on a particular day, such as a birthday party, or to indicate a regularly scheduled event. For instance, if your child has karate on Wednesdays and you indicate it on his timetable, then indicate the information on the calendar as well. Any kind of reinforcement is helpful.

The calendar can also be used to prepare your child for a parent's trip away. Indicate the days you will be gone with a symbol of the trip (perhaps a picture of a plane, your destination, or the person you will visit). Be sure to indicate the day you will be returning—that will be the most crucial information to your child.

One traditional and effective method for teaching calendar skills to typical children is the use of sequenced visual patterns. These can be as simple as ABC patterns or seed-sprout-tree; the patterns can become more complex as your child's understanding increases with time. (See page 27 for sequencing examples.)

To teach your child calendar skills, we suggest that you take a blank calendar (preferably a dry-erase marker board of substantial size) and write the days of the week at the top. Use the pictures on page 201 or make your own to create a simple sequenced pattern. Have your child write today's date on the picture and put it on the calendar. As the pattern progresses, your child will recognize which picture comes next in the sequence. This process helps your child integrate the calendar days and dates and understand the passage of time.

You can often use theme-based pictures that correspond with events that are taking place in a given month. For example, if the month is October find a sequence of pictures that evoke a harvest theme. This will help your child integrate his experience with what the rest of the world is experiencing.

Play is an activity natural to animals, perhaps to all living things. It may be the simplest and purest expression of life itself, of the delight living beings take in the sheer fact of their own existence.

—LAWRENCE KIMMEL

SAMPLE CALENDAR

See page 24 for explanations; see Part Three for sequencing cutouts.

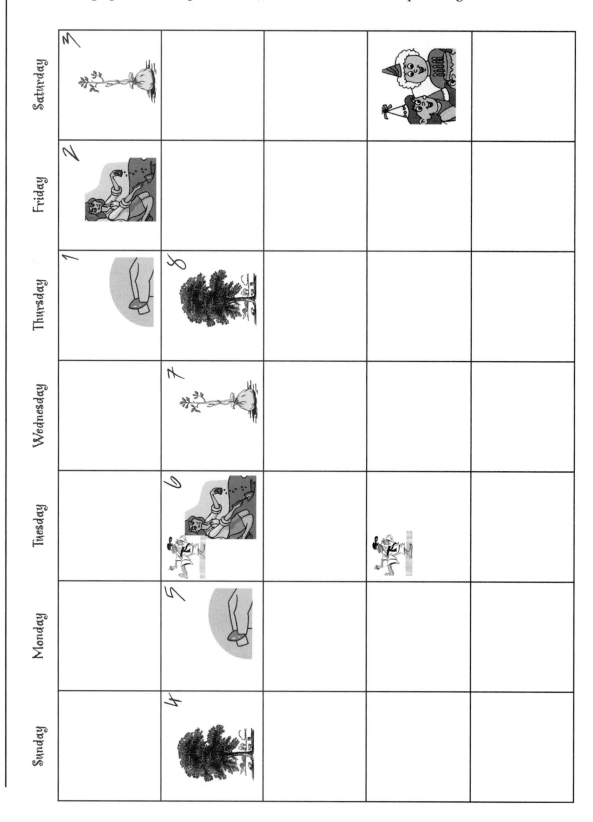

SEQUENCING EXAMPLES (See Part Three for cutouts)

SHAPE PATTERNS

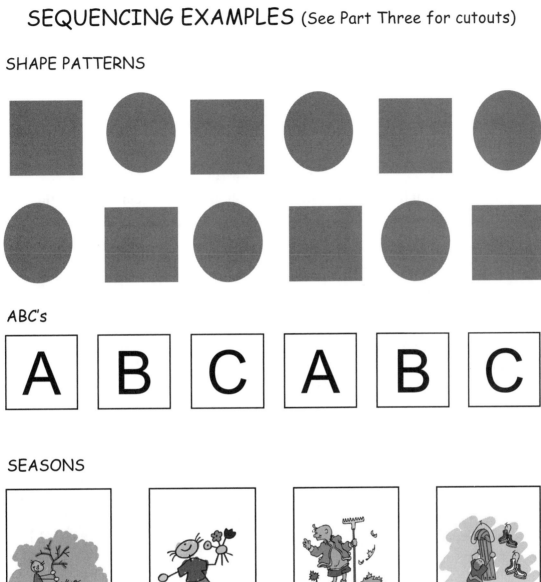

ABC's

| A | B | C | A | B | C |

SEASONS

spring   summer   autumn   winter

GROWTH

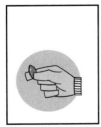 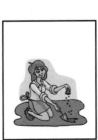 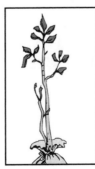 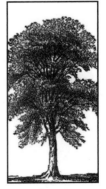 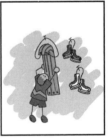 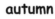

seed   planting   sapling   tree

Visual Cue Box

Another way to help your child cope with what's going on is to create a box filled with images that will help her visualize events. Cut out magazine pictures, download appropriate online images, take photos with your camera, cut out box labels from your child's favorite foods, and put them all in the box. Use your imagination!

When you have to go to the barber shop for a haircut, pull out the visuals you've clipped for this trip: a picture of the car, seatbelts, a barber shop, a person getting a haircut—whatever you think will help your child with this adventure.

At the beginning of the day you can make a game of finding the visuals that match events on your daily schedule. Put them into a small notebook (a small photo album works great) and take them along with you.

> Keep the "Visual Cue Box" accessible so your child can use it when she wants to communicate something to you.

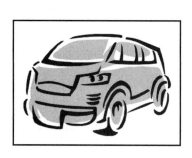
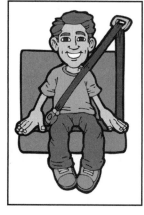
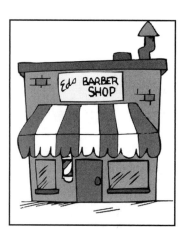
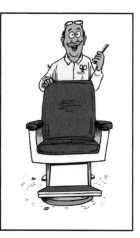
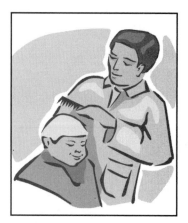

Fridge Central

We've discovered that the refrigerator can be used as an information center for your child. My wife divided our refrigerator into squares, with a copy of Eli's daily schedule affixed with magnets or tape in one section. Another section might display a picture of an upcoming afternoon errand. The third section often shows a picture of a family member or friend who is going to be visiting later in the day. One section always has a picture of where Mom or Dad is at the moment so that when my son asks, "Where's Mama?" I can easily refer to the picture as a way of reinforcing the verbal answer that I've given him (countless times).

You can use the refrigerator as a location where your child knows she can go to get information. We call it "fridge central."

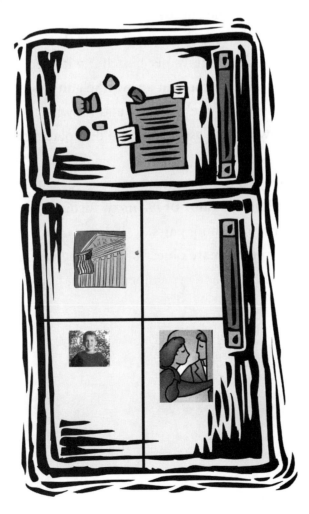

Daily Recap

As discussed earlier, children on the autistic spectrum can experience difficulty with the concept of time and the sequencing of events. In an effort to help your child relate to what has occurred during his day, it is always helpful to have a recap that night. Not only will this process work on developing the concept of sequencing the past, it will also help in connecting to the present and the future.

The use of visual cues is very effective in helping to solidify your child's memory. The game on page 31 can help your child relive visually the events of the day. The setup is very similar to TicTacToe. Your child must match three pictures in a row of events that occurred during the day. You can create a variety of ways for your child to discover the cards, depending on her level of development.

Set up a stack of the cutout cards face up or down. (See pages 173, 175 and 177.) Pick from the top of the pile. If the card is something your child did that day, have her match it with the picture on the board. When you have three in a row, the game is over. (Note: If she eats three meals a day, she'll always end up with three in a row.) After a three-in-a-row match, assist your child in placing the events in chronological order.

Another way to use the cutout cards is to scatter them on the floor face-down and play a game of *memory*, turning over cards two at a time in search of matching pairs.

Of course, the ultimate object of the game is not to win but to have your child relive and remember what happened during his day.

Children on the autistic spectrum "do not understand ambiguity or double meanings and take every-thing literally. They are confused by sarcasm or irony, which should be avoided when talking to them."

—LORNA WING, M.D.

WHAT I DID TODAY—
THREE IN A ROW BINGO

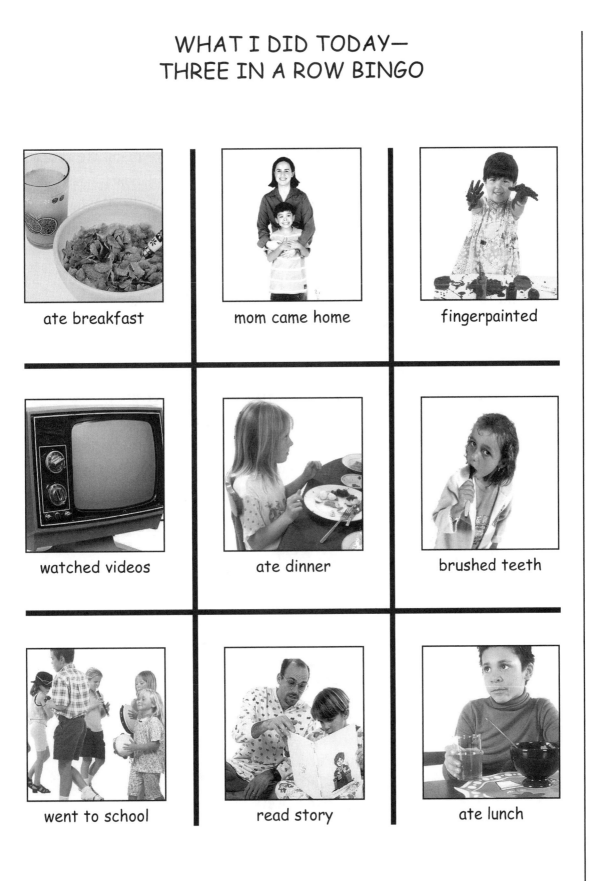

ate breakfast	mom came home	fingerpainted
watched videos	ate dinner	brushed teeth
went to school	read story	ate lunch

Telling Stories

A time-tested method of assisting children with autism to relate to the world is telling them their own true stories. If you think about it, that is what we are doing when we are creating schedules for them. We are telling them the story of what they are going to do for the day.

Your story can be revisited at the end of the day as well. Did the day go as planned? Did all the things on the schedule happen? What was the same, what was different? This revisiting of the events of the day is a wonderful way to help your child develop the sense of time and place that is so crucial to being integrated in the world.

As your child gets older the need for schedules may diminish, but the use of stories can still be effective as a tool for discussing how particular events during the day made him feel.

You can even use some language arts strategies for creating these stories by building on a word and extending the thoughts outward. Having your child connect the words and thoughts will also be an entry into his emotional experience of the event. This is called a story web.

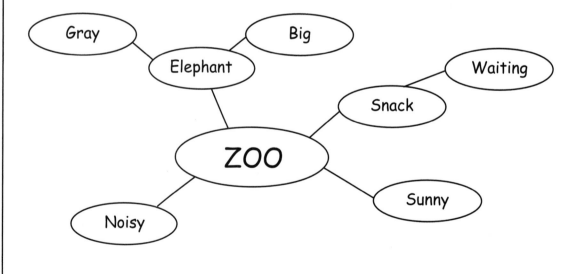

Story web

3

SELF-CARE— TEACHING THE BASICS

Regardless of your child's exceptionalities, perhaps the most important aspect of her education is learning how to navigate through life as a child and ultimately as an adult. Without basic life skills, the exceptional child will be lost in a large and sometimes frightening world without a compass. Your ultimate goal is to help your child become as independent as possible and live her life to the fullest extent.

Helping your child experience independence is possibly the most monumental job you'll face. It is certainly the most rewarding, as we discover when that independence is achieved— even when it comes to the smallest of tasks.

Self-care is the ability to care for your own basic needs. Self-care skills are essential in helping your child to create an independent life. Your child's mastery of tasks such as dressing, bathing, brushing teeth, learning how to use money, and fixing a snack will make life easier for all members of the family. Your child will feel a wonderful sense of autonomy and you'll be relieved of some of your daily duties.

What follows are a few suggestions for making self-care a reality.

Getting Dressed

**Backward
chaining:**

"Teaching a
task begin-
ning with the
last step,
then the
next to last
step, and so
on, so that
the child is
aware of
completing a
task success-
fully."

—LORNA
WING, M.D.

Getting dressed independently is an important part of self-care. It seems simple enough to learn; children who are not impaired learn this skill primarily by imitation. Your child will probably have a more difficult time learning the process. Think about it. Not only do you have choices to make—what clothes to wear if it is cold or hot outside, which apparel is appropriate for the occasion—but you need to know how to put them on in the proper sequence. Then you need to figure out which is the front of the garment and whether it's inside out. Not so easy after all, is it?

Never fear, your child can learn to dress himself. His best chance to do this is through direct experience. One method of teaching this skill is called backward chaining. This method breaks a process down into small steps. Begin with the last step first, having your child *master* it before going on to the step that goes before it. For instance, perhaps you are teaching your child to put on socks. Begin by putting the sock almost all the way onto his foot, pulling it over toe and heel. Teach your child to pull the sock up the rest of the way. The next step is teaching him to pull the sock over his heel; then to put the toe into

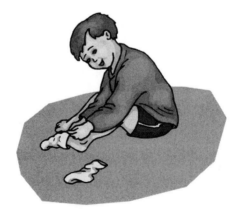

the sock, etc. Be patient: it may take a long time for each step to be mastered.

Once your child has learned how to put on each article of clothing, it is time to teach her the proper order for dressing. Imagine if you put your pants on, then your underwear. How funny would that be? Use humor to help your child recognize the *incorrect* order for dressing. Next place the clothes in front of your child in the correct order so that she can learn how to do this.

Another method of teaching your child to dress is to manipulate her hands as you help dress her. For example, when buttoning a blouse, physically guide her through the movements necessary. (Try to select clothing with large buttons and other easy fasteners.) Her fingers may feel limp at first, but persevere—after a while she will be buttoning the garment herself. Be sure to give her positive feedback every time she does something right.

Sometimes, in this hectic world, you don't have time to wait for your child to dress himself. Still, try to remember that the more you do for your child the less he is interested in doing for himself. So give yourself plenty of time in the morning—and if putting on all the clothes is too daunting a task for your child, give yourself a break and pick one or two items that are your child's responsibility to put on while you do the rest. When you're in a hurry, reinforcers can also help speed up the process by motivating your child. (See pages 76–78.)

USING HUMOR TO CREATE PROBLEM-SOLVING ADVENTURES FOR YOUR CHILD

Make getting dressed fun, not a chore.

When Getting Dressed:

- Put socks on your child's hands instead of his feet.
- Put two socks on one foot.
- Put your child's shirt on his feet and legs.
- Give him your shoes to wear.

Using these ideas to make him laugh, have him tell you what's wacky. This opens up opportunities for communication and fun!

GETTING DRESSED MATCHING GAME

(Draw a line from each piece of clothing to the part
of the body where you wear it.)

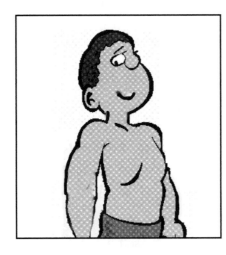
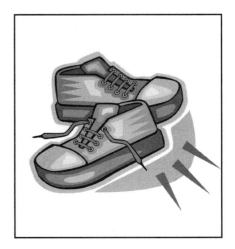

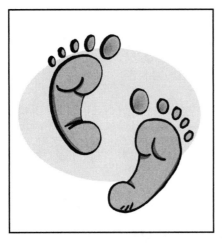
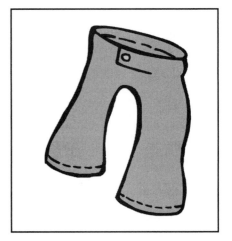

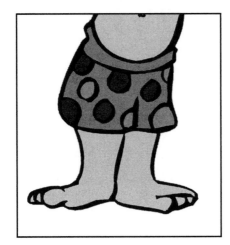
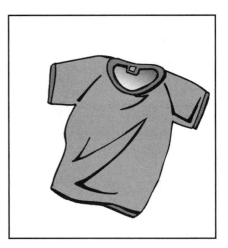

Toothbrushing

Dental hygiene is a challenge. If you listed all the separate steps that go into brushing teeth, you would be amazed: entering the bathroom, finding the toothbrush, picking up the brush, rinsing the brush, finding the toothpaste, taking off the cap, squeezing the tube—and we haven't even started brushing the teeth yet!

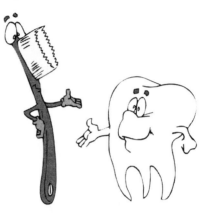

How to achieve dental hygiene? Backward chaining (see page 81) can help. Don't expect your child to be able to handle every step of tooth brushing right from the beginning: begin by teaching the final steps, and work backward as your child masters each step.

Once my son was brushing his own teeth, I discovered a terrific method for reminding him what to do. I made up a different funny sound for each area that needed brushing. First I had my boy smile, and as he was moving the brush back and forth I made an "eeeeeee" sound. Then, when it was time for him to open wide and brush the back teeth, the sound changed to "aaaahhhhhhh."

EEEEEEEEEEE AAAAAHHHHHHHH
EEEEEEEEEEE AAAAAHHHHHHHH
EEEEEEEEEEE AAAAAHHHHHHHH

My son still tends to chew on his brush sometimes, but as soon as I prompt him with the EEEEEEEEEEE AAAAAHHHHHHHH sounds he remembers to start moving his brush back and forth and then open his mouth and brush those back teeth.

You might also consider having your child brush her teeth while she's in the bathtub. Kids who enjoy the tub as much as my boy does tend to be very relaxed there.

You can also create a step-by-step written or visual list for brushing teeth. Here's an example:

BRUSHING TEETH

1. Take off toothpaste cap

2. Get toothbrush

3. Put toothpaste on toothbrush

4. Put cap back on toothpaste

5. Set timer to 15 seconds

6. Brush front teeth until the timer rings

7. Set timer to 15 seconds

8. Brush right side of teeth until the timer rings

9. Set timer to 15 seconds

10. Brush left side of teeth until the timer rings

11. Set timer to 15 seconds

12. Brush inside of teeth until the timer rings

13. Rinse mouth

14. Rinse toothbrush

15. Put toothbrush away

Bathing

Learning self-care will obviously involve understanding proper hygiene. For younger children on the autistic spectrum, taking a bath can be an opportunity to develop imaginative play. On the other hand, when children hate the tub, bathtime can be a nightmare for parents who want their child to be clean!

Bathing is an area where suggestions for typical children come in handy—even if they're not quite age appropriate for your child. Bathtubs can be safety hazards if you are not paying attention. Remember:

- be aware of the water temperature—not too hot...and brrrr, not too cold
- place a rubber mat (or an old towel if your child doesn't like the feel of rubber) on the bottom of the tub to prevent slipping
- teach your child not to touch the taps (see safety images on page 194) so that he won't burn himself
- keep the water shallow
- never leave your child unsupervised

If your child really hates the bath, you might use a hand shower in an empty tub to rinse her off. Many kids really hate shampooing—this can be kept to a minimum if your child's hair is cut short. (Of course, then you have to deal with hair cutting. Decide which is more difficult!)

Bath toys inspire games. Ask questions that stimulate creative thinking and let your child initiate stories. For example, if your child pushes a toy boat under the water, point out that everyone on the boat must be getting wet. Ask whether they are enjoying swimming in the tub. Choose comments that invite a response.

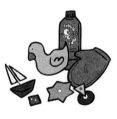

Eventually you will want to teach your child the steps of soaping, rinsing and drying off. This activity lends itself well to play. Have your child help wash the car, and talk about how

Handwashing is an important detail to introduce to your child. Frequent handwashing will prevent the spread of germs. Ahhchoo!

you use soap to wash, the hose to rinse and towels to dry the car. You can have your child practice washing a doll. Use your creativity to come up with playful learning opportunities.

If your child is fearful of bathing, consider the story of a child named James who was afraid of the bathtub, which Lorna Wing related in *The Autistic Spectrum*:

Maria, an au pair *living with the family who was good with children, popped him into a bath on the first day she arrived, unaware of his fear. His astonished mother heard happy giggles and splashes and found her child enjoying his first bath in years as if he had one every day. In this case, it seems that the child was helped by the fact that Maria was not anticipating fear, whereas his parents had grown accustomed to it.*

James' parents also learned from the experience and were much more confident and successful in dealing with other, similar problems that occurred. It is interesting that Maria, who arrived knowing hardly any English, developed a close rapport with James because, as she explained, they both had a language problem and both were, so to speak, strangers in a strange land.

Fixing a Snack

"Mama, I need some juice. Mama, I need some cottage cheese."

These are words that echo through our house, sometimes at an alarming rate. What to do? Create an opportunity for your child to help himself and to have a successful experience doing it. Don't forget to make it a situation where *you* don't have to clean up a big mess if things don't go well. How can you do that?

- Create shelf space in a low cupboard for your child's snack needs.
- Fill that space with plates and bowls that will not shatter if accidentally dropped.
- Create a space in the fridge where your child can reach her favorite snack items.
- Put those items in containers that are easy for your child to handle with success.

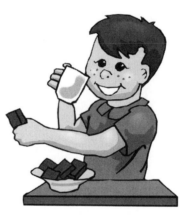

As with many of the self-care skills, one of the best teaching strategies is backward chaining. (See page 81.) Help your child master each step, starting at the *end* of the task. For example, begin by fixing him a snack and having him carry it to the table himself. The next time, have him put the crackers on the plate and carry it to the table. In the end, he'll be able to get out the crackers and fix the snack himself. Remember to praise him when he accomplishes a task!

Begin as early as you can when teaching your child self-care. Otherwise he might resist any change in his daily habits. If he depends on you for everything, he might not have the desire to take care of himself as best he can.

My Room

Another way to help your child achieve independence is to label her personal space, enabling her to find items and put them away. Managing her own belongings will give your child more freedom. The labels also develop her communication skills. Finding the right place to put her clothes is a fun way to learn matching skills, as well as a way to give your life some semblance of order.

Here are a few suggestions

◘ Label her dresser with words or pictures of the items that belong in each drawer—undies, socks, pants, shirts, etc.

◘ Label shelves or containers for toys, activity tools and other belongings. Don't forget your Visual Cue Box.

You might consider labeling other areas of the house to help your child find things she might need. (Don't go overboard!)

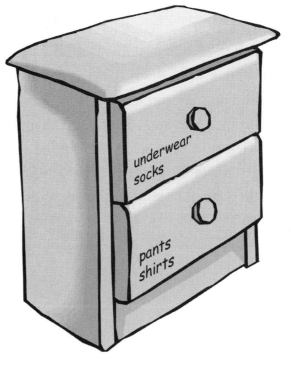

Telling Time

Reading clocks is a skill that most typical children start to learn in their first-grade curriculum. Even for typical kids, it's a challenge to distinguish the big hand from the little hand and to know the significance of each. Reading the minutes is even more complex, especially since those numbers aren't found on the clock face.

So why should your child tackle this skill? For one thing, our society is very time-conscious. How else will we know when *SpongeBob SquarePants* is on television, or what time Dad will be home from the office? In addition to being a life skill, learning to tell time helps your child feel more secure when following his timetable, especially when he is older and needs to be self-reliant.

On page 219 is a clock template to help your child master telling time. You can create clock hands in several ways. You can laminate the picture of the clock and then use a wipe-off marker to draw the hands (probably the best way) or you can assist your child in cutting hands out of construction paper and using a brad to attach them.

So how do you go about teaching this skill? Start by drilling the hours. Begin with the hands on 12. Once your child knows 12 o'clock, move on to 1 o'clock, 2 o'clock and so on. After he masters the hours, move on to half past the hour, and then quarter past. Learning the minutes will be easier if your child can count by fives. (See the number grid on page 166.) You can also write the minutes on the outside of your clock as we have done in the example in Part Two.

Here's one game I played with my son:

Using a funny little voice I said, "The little hand is the hand that announces the hour. Wherever the little hand is pointing, that is the hour of the day."

Using a funny deep voice I said, "The big hand tells you the minutes."

In a funny little voice: "The time is 4 o'clock..."

Changing to the deep voice: "...and 15 minutes."

Consider using an old discarded clock as a teaching "tool" for learning time.

SAMPLE CLOCKS AND HANDS

Some children who can tell time by the clock become obsessed with time and demand that everything happen at the exact time stated. In that case, you need to be careful about saying something as innocuous as "We'll leave in two minutes."

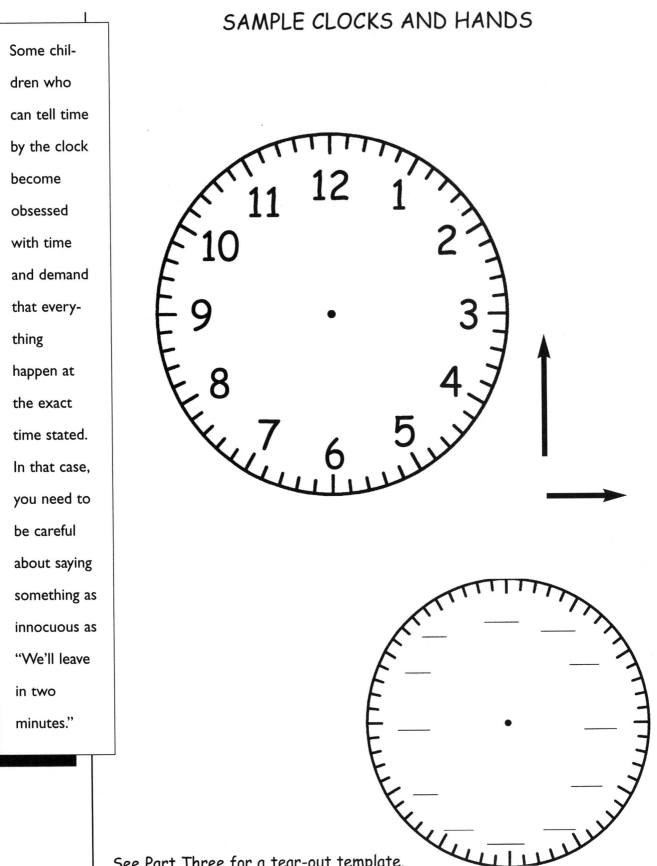

See Part Three for a tear-out template.

4

IN THE WORLD

Unless we are hermits in a mountain cave, we all have to function in the world. That is even true for a child on the autistic spectrum. Yet for such a child, being out and about can be confusing and scary. You know that you can't keep your child separated from the confusion; families need to function in as normal a fashion as possible. So it becomes important for you to map out strategies that make each outing tolerable—and yes, even fun.

Again, planning is the key to creating such successful ventures. Detailing in words and pictures where you are going, what will be happening, how long the trip will last, and—most importantly—the fact that you will return home, will help your child feel more secure.

What will make outings easier for both you and your child? Here are some of our ideas:

- Keep transitions in mind. Before you leave, give your child enough warning to get ready on time, and give him a heads-up before you plan to return home (if he hasn't already grabbed your hand and demanded to return home "NOW").
- It is best to keep your first trips short and not too far from home so that if your child becomes too stressed you can easily return.
- Bring along familiar toys or belongings and snacks—they can be a comfort or a welcome distraction.
- Constantly remind your child what is coming next.

Our family has found the "countdown" to be an effective method for dealing with transitions. Before the appointed time, start letting your child know that the next event (leaving, arriving, activity, etc.) will happen soon. You can start at 20 minutes before and count down in five-minute intervals. At five minutes start counting down by minutes. Don't worry if you need to adjust the real time, because the ultimate goal is to calm your child by keeping him informed.

Be sure to communicate clearly: "Elijah, ten more minutes and then it is time to stop playing on the computer."

Alleviating the abruptness will give the child time to prepare for the inevitable change.

We have provided information in this section to help make trips to the doctor, the dentist, even the grocery store, easier. This kind of preparation may sound like a lot of work, but it's a lot easier to prepare your child for what is happening than to manage your child once she has gone out of control.

> When setting out on any expedition, it should be made clear that it will end in a return home or other base.
>
> —LORNA WING, M.D.

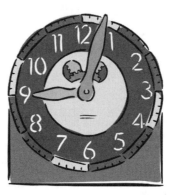

Countdown!

Why Is He Acting Like That?

Okay. You've taken your child out in the world, where he'll come face to face with people who do not understand his behavior. Many will stare at him or shake their heads in disgust if he is acting out. Some people will even have the gall to call you on your parenting techniques.

Short of hanging a sign on your child's back that reads "I'm not misbehaving. I'm a Special Needs Child. Leave us alone," what can you do?

We've provided a sheet on the basic facts about autism for you. Feel free to give this to family members, friends, neighbors, doctors, dentists, hairdressers—anyone you can think of who will benefit from this knowledge. We hope it will make them more accepting of your child, and make visits with them easier for all of you.

We've also devised a little card that you can find in Part Three if you are tired of the stares. It will probably disarm the person who is irritating you, and educate her at the same time.

My child is on the
Autistic Spectrum.

For more information about autism
go to:
www.autism-society.org.

Basic Facts about Autism

The following definition is from the Autism Society of America: Autism is a severely incapacitating lifelong developmental disability that typically appears during the first three years of life. It occurs in approximately fifteen out of every 10,000 births and is four times more common in boys than girls. It has been found throughout the world in families of all racial, ethnic and social backgrounds. No known factors in the psychological environment of a child have been shown to cause autism. The symptoms are caused by physical disorders of the brain. They include:

1. Disturbances in the rate of appearance of physical, social and language skills.
2. Abnormal responses to sensations. Any one or a combination of senses or responses are affected: sight, hearing, touch, pain, balance, smell, taste and the way a child holds his body.
3. Speech and language are absent or delayed, while specific thinking capabilities might be present.
4. Abnormal ways of relating to people, objects and events.

SIGNS OF AUTISM

- No pointing by one year
- No babbling by one year; no single words by 16 months; no two-word phrases by 24 months
- Loss of language skills at any time
- No pretend playing
- Little interest in making friends
- Extremely short attention span
- No response when called by name; indifference to others
- Little or no eye contact
- Repetitive body movement, such as hand flapping or rocking
- Intense tantrums
- Fixations on a single object, such as a spinning fan
- Unusually strong resistance to changes in routines
- Over-sensitivity to certain sounds, textures or smells

A Sample Letter for Your Hairdresser, Shoe Store Clerk or Anyone You Feel Is Appropriate

(Note: You can add your child's name to make it more personal. See page 213 in Part Three for a sample to copy.)

Dear_____,

    This is a letter of introduction. My child will be visiting your establishment soon. She is a special needs child on the autistic spectrum. As you may know, interactions with strangers are very stressful for such a child and I am trying to make this visit as easy as possible for all of us.

    If you would like to know more about autism prior to this visit, I would be most happy to send you pertinent information. You can also find information on the following website: www.autism-society.org. My child has a difficult time expressing her feelings, and any supplementary knowledge you have may make it easier for you to communicate with her.

    We look forward to meeting you.

Sincerely,

A Sample Letter
for Your Doctor or Dentist

Grand-
parents,
aunts and
uncles often
establish a
special bond
with their
grandchild,
niece or
nephew.
When possi-
ble, use them
as a resource
for emo-
tional and
practical
help.

(Note: You can add your child's name to make it more personal. See page 211 in Part Three for a sample to copy.)

Dear_____,

    This is a letter of introduction. My child will soon be visiting your office. He is a special needs child on the autistic spectrum. As you may know, interactions with strangers are very stressful for such a child. I am trying to make this visit easy for all of us.

    Is it possible for us to visit your office prior to the scheduled appointment so that my child can become familiar with the surroundings as well as with you and your staff? This may make the actual appointment more successful. I realize that you are very busy, and I will understand if this would not work out.

    If you would like to know more about autism prior to this visit, I would be happy to send you pertinent information. You can also find information on the following website: www.autism-society.org.

    My child has a difficult time expressing his feelings, and any supplementary knowledge you have may make it easier for you to communicate with him.

    One aspect of life that is particularly difficult for children on the autistic spectrum is their lack of a concept of time. Having to wait in a waiting room is difficult for any child. It is even more so for mine. If possible, I would like to arrange for us to be your first appointment of the day. This will ensure there will be less disruption to your office.

    If an anesthetic needs to be used, please note that it may excite my child, since children on the autistic spectrum often respond to sedatives in a contrary fashion.

    Please share this letter with your office staff so that they will be prepared for our visit as well.

    We look forward to meeting you.

Sincerely,

Visiting Friends and Family

Trips to other people's homes can afford you valuable "adult time," as well as offer some emotional support. It is important to keep up with family ties and not neglect your friendships. But we know that this is not easy!

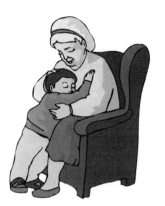

Making these visits work involves preparation. (That word keeps cropping up, doesn't it?) Here are a few suggestions:

■ Create a list of things you should bring. Don't forget special food, toys, favorite books, videos and a change of clothes.

■ Talk to the people you are going to visit. Explain to them that you may have to focus much of your attention on your child. Suggest they think of it as if you were bringing a two-year-old to visit—you wouldn't leave her unsupervised.

■ Teach your child the name of the people she will be visiting and, if you can, prompt her to say hello on arrival and goodbye when leaving.

■ When you arrive, acquaint your child with the house. Show her the bathroom.

■ Keep visits short and trust that in time, over repeated visits, your visits will become longer and more relaxed as your child grows accustomed to the surroundings.

AN EXAMPLE: GOING TO GRANDMA'S HOUSE

■ Paste a photograph of Grandma in your child's workbook, and if possible, a picture of the house where she lives.

■ Describe the last time you visited Grandma and some of the activities you did together.

■ Tell your child how you will travel to Grandma's—by car, plane, train, boat or bus—and how you will return home.

■ Talk about what you plan to do at Grandma's: eat a meal, play in the yard, watch a video.

■ When you return from the outing, write down what you did. If you took photos, paste them in your child's workbook and review them the next day and then again before your next visit. You could even create a special memory book for each trip.

Visiting the Doctor

Let's face it: no one really enjoys going to the doctor. It is a visit that makes almost everyone anxious. Blood pressures go up, pulse rates increase. So how can you make it easier for your child to do something none of us enjoy doing?

Laying the groundwork is the key to making doctor visits work. Giving your child the necessary information ahead of time will ready her for the impending appointment. Part Two includes a story about going to the doctor's office to help you with this preparation. We recommend you and your child read through the story a number of times to familiarize your child with what will be happening.

Informing the doctor and the office staff about your child is also helpful. This is where the letter on page 50 will come in handy. Make certain you schedule the visit for the most convenient time. Try to be the first or last person to see the doctor, if possible. Come prepared with materials that will interest your child while you wait, unless you believe she will be more content to sit quietly.

If it is time for an inoculation, or if your child is ill and may need a shot, it's best to prepare your child for that possibility. Teaching him relaxation techniques and reassuring words ahead of time might make having a needle stuck into him less threatening. Breathing techniques, such as taking deep breaths and slowly blowing the air out, can often calm an anxious child, or at least distract him.

Be aware that some children do not react negatively to medical procedures: They are fascinated by such goings on and may be detached from the anxiety you might be feeling. Remember, your child is unique and you should try to plan accordingly. You might want to contact the office ahead of time to find out what the doctor is scheduling for this visit and create a short list for your child to review. The list could be visual or written, depending on her abilities. See the following page for an example.

Sample: This is an example of a one-page sheet you can take on a visit to the doctor. It will make your child feel more secure to know what will be happening next.

WHAT'S GOING TO HAPPEN AT THE DOCTOR'S OFFICE

Time to visit Dr. Jones

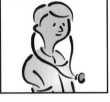

Sit in the waiting room

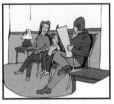

Go into the examining room and be measured

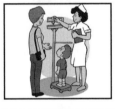

Be checked by Dr. Jones

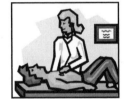

Get a shot and then get a sticker as a reward

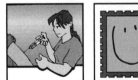

Go to Blarney's for a lemonade treat

Go home

Visiting the Dentist

It is important for your child to feel as comfortable as possible when visiting the dentist. Some dentists have found that incorporating humor into their practice will put children at ease, making the task of dental hygiene easier for both the dentist and your child. For example, "We have to use a light because your mouth doesn't have windows!"

You might want to set up an appointment (in person or over the phone) with your child's dentist to talk about your child's special needs. The same traits that you would look for in a behaviorist or therapist might apply to your dentist as well.

- Does the dentist have a personality (lots of affect!) that works well with children?
- Does the dentist use humor to help put the child at ease?
- Does the dentist have a TV that the child can watch during the procedure? If she does, bring a favorite video!
- Does the dentist use the "Tell, Show and Do" technique? This helps to desensitize the child to the anxiety-provoking stimuli.
    1) Tell the child what is going to happen.
    2) Show the child the equipment that will be used.
    3) Do the procedure.

See page 211 for a sample letter to send to your child's dentist.

Grocery Shopping

Running errands with a child with autism can be a journey laden with difficulty. Even a trip to the grocery store can be daunting. My son does not have very good lane sense, and so we are always on the lookout for those moments when he might inadvertently crash into some unsuspecting shopper.

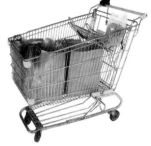

He does love to participate, though. One of the ways that we have found to alleviate his anxiety is to include him in the process. He reads, so we can offer him a typed list of some of the items to be removed from the shelf.

If your child cannot read yet, make up a card for each item by cutting and taping a label or picture to a four-by-six index card. Write the names of the items on the index cards and arrange the index cards in the order you would come across them during your excursion through the store.

If you need to, you can use the backward chaining method to include him in the shopping trip. (See page 81.) Start by handing your child the item to be placed in the cart. After he masters that step, move on to having him remove the item from the shelf and placing into the cart. The final step is to have him locate the item on the shelf, remove it, and place it in the cart. Remember to have him master each step in the backward chain before you move to the next step.

Don't forget the milk!

Sensory overload can occur in even the most mundane places—such as the grocery store.

Going to the Movies

The movie theater can be a place of great fun or great anxiety. Many children with autism suffer from sensory overload in certain environments, and the movie theater is often one of them. Theater sound systems are designed to create a very loud and exciting experience for those with typical hearing, but what of the person with autism whose hearing is extra sensitive? The light from the screen can also be extra bright in the context of a darkened theater.

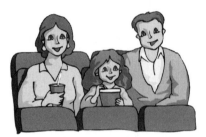

How can you create a more pleasurable experience for your child? Of course, the first and most important thing to figure out is…does your child want to go to the movies? If so, you might try some of the methods that we use to help our son enjoy his experience.

1) Preparation, preparation, preparation. Do your best to plan ahead and make transitions smooth. If you can, prepay for your tickets so that you don't have to wait in long ticket lines. There is usually a small service charge for tickets purchased over the phone or internet, but it is a small price to pay for peace of mind.

2) Find ways to make your child's sensory experience more pleasant. We use a pair of stereo headphones to help reduce the noise level. Go at your child's pace. For the longest time our son kept his hands over his eyes at the movies. But now he sits calmly with his headphones on and enjoys the movie on his own terms.

3) Get to the theater early, before the trailers start. This will allow for an easier transition than walking into an already-darkened theater. Give your child some choices about where to sit. Try to guide him to pick a seat close to the aisle, so that if he needs to take a break it will be easy to move.

4) Nowadays many theaters have video games in the lobby. If your child likes to play these games, you can take a break from the feature in the lobby. Be sure your child understands that you will be going back to the movie after a certain amount of time.

5) Let go of your desire to watch the whole movie. Your child might not be able to sit through a whole feature—or she might not want to. It may be disheartening not to take full advantage of your paid admission, but you will feel better if you reconcile those thoughts before the show starts. You can always rent the movie later and see the end if *you* were enthralled.

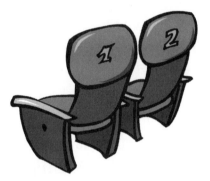

Amusing Parks

Going to an amusement park can be a wonderful experience or a disaster from hell. There are a few things you can do to help the experience fall more on the wonderful side.

1) Find out if the park offers special assistance passes. These are invaluable for the child who has difficulty standing in the long lines that are fairly routine at popular parks. Generally people in wheelchairs or on crutches use these passes, and they enable your group to enter a ride at the exit and thus bypass the long lines. Make sure to take a printed diagnosis from the doctor's office in case the park requires verification of your child's special needs. Also be aware that some parks place limits on the number of people who can be in your group entering the ride from the exit. Because these passes are becoming more commonplace, there is sometimes a bit of a wait at the exits for certain rides. Still, the lines are always shorter than the regular lines.

2) Take it slow. If your child finds a ride that she really likes (our favorite is the Casey Jr. Train at Disneyland) then spend some time there first and use it as a positive reinforcer. If your child knows that she will be coming back to her favorite ride she will be more willing to explore other areas of the park.

3) Plan out what areas you will be visiting in the park and create an itinerary with your child. Most of the parks have internet sites with maps, and these can be printed out and used to great effect to help your child *know* what will be happening on this exciting adventure. Be sure to remember that plans can change for various reasons. With that in mind...

4) Look for the quiet areas of the park. There are sure to be some spots where fewer people are congregating, and these places can be a great refuge from the sensory overload that comes with the territory at an amusement park.

5) If your child is a picky eater, remember to bring her favorite snacks, as they will probably not be available inside the park. Most park food is fried and filled with sugar, so it is wise to bring some

Humor is the healthy way of feeling a "distance" between one's self and the problem, a way of standing off and looking at one's problem with perspective.

—ROLLO MAY

nutritious snacks that can be eaten in one of those quiet places you found when scouting around. A quiet place may be a much more favorable location for eating than a table inside a noisy restaurant, especially when your child is in sensory overload and too excited to sit still.

6) As with a trip to the movies, let go of any expectations you might have about the length of your stay. All of the inflexibility that a child with autism sometimes carries must be met with the flexibility of a contortionist on the part of the parent. Listen to your child's reactions and gauge when it is time to leave so that you can depart with a positive experience.

7) After you have come home and relaxed a bit, take another trip, this time using pictures taken from the day. (Remember to bring a camera!) With the photos, create a few pages of memories to place in your child's binder. Use these pages as visual aids for engaging your child in conversation. Ask about his favorite rides or his favorite place in the park. These high-affect "trips" can be used to elicit wonderful conversations with your child and also help to prepare for the next time your family takes a trip to the amusement park.

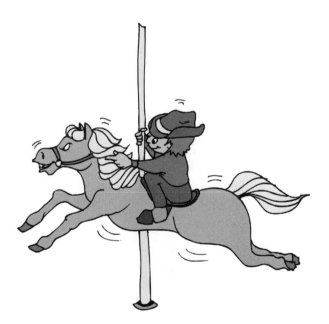

Helping around the House

You can help your child become a part of the world by strengthening her sense of being a valued part of your family. One way to do this is to create chores that she is capable of completing. Not only do chores give her a sense of place in the family, they help build self-esteem.

Having your child water plants in the garden can be a fun way to learn that plants need water to survive and gives your child an opportunity to play with water. Eventually, it will also mean one less thing for you to do. Taking out the garbage is another task that can be broken down into small steps a child can learn over time. Be sure to praise your child after he has completed each step.

But be aware: while many children with autism like to be praised, there are a few who become angry or contrary if praised for anything. This may be because they dislike being picked out as different. If your child is that way, be careful to avoid verbal approval. Try effective non-verbal signs such as a thumbs-up or smile.

What follows are some simple tasks that your child might try, along with instructions for helping your child accomplish them. They will help your child feel a part of the family.

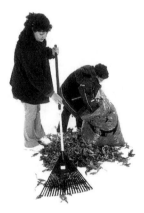

SETTING THE TABLE

Let's learn the names of the utensils we use to eat with.

Here's a knife.

This is a fork.

Here's a spoon.

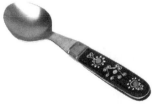

What else do we use on the table?

A glass.
What do we put in your glass?

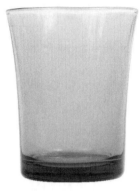

Napkins.
What do we use napkins for?

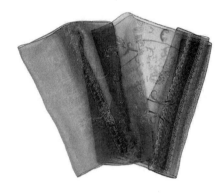

Here are the salt
and pepper shakers.

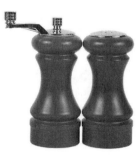

CHORES

You can help your child with chores by creating lists and/or visuals for various tasks.

Here are some examples:

THINGS TO DO TO CLEAN YOUR BEDROOM

- Put clothes away

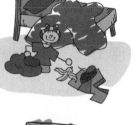

- Put toys in toy box

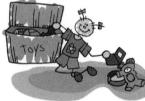

- Put dirty clothes in hamper

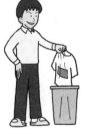

WATERING THE PLANTS

- Get watering can
- Put water in watering can
- Sprinkle water on plants
- Make sure can is empty
- Put watering can back on shelf

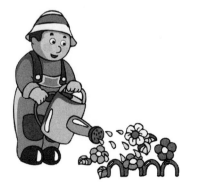

Doing a chore helps your child feel like she contributes to the family. Completing the task builds self-esteem.

Money Counts

Learning about money is a good opportunity to review numbers with your child.

One of the most important steps to your child's future independence is learning about money and its varying values. Included in your child's workbook are several money worksheets to help him learn the amounts.

There are sheets to help familiarize your child with the different names and values of the coins and paper bills. Also included are sheets for playing matching games with the various denominations.

You can help your child practice money values by setting up a "store" in your house. Indicate the price for each item visually, with a picture of the coins needed, or by writing the amounts in cents if your child can read.

Make the store contents fun. The items "for sale" should be things your child wants and enjoys. This will make the process of learning much more enjoyable.

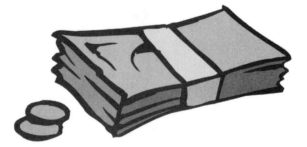

COINS

When you go into the store you need money to buy things. Sometimes you pay with coins. Let's learn our coins.

One penny. A penny is brown.
You need lots of pennies to buy something.
1 cent

1

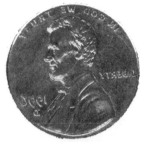

One nickel.
A nickel is silver.
It is the fattest coin.
5 cents

1 2 3 4 5

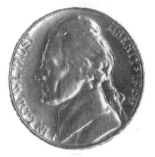

One dime. A dime is the smallest silver coin.
10 cents

1 2 3 4 5
6 7 8 9 10

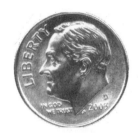

One quarter. A quarter is silver and bigger than a nickel.
25 cents

1 2 3 4 5 6 7 8 9
10 11 12 13 14 15
16 17 18 19 20 21
22 23 24 25

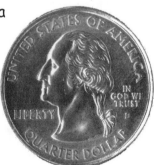

PAPER MONEY

When you go into the store you need money to buy things. You pay with coins some of the time, but you will use paper money for most things. Paper money is called "bills." Let's learn our bills.

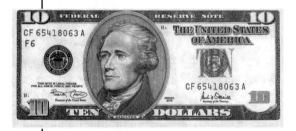

One-dollar bill. Dollars are used a lot.

1

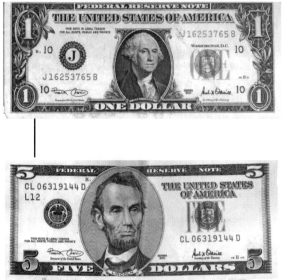

Five-dollar bill. A five-dollar bill is the same as five one-dollar bills.

1 2 3 4 5

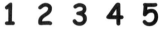

Ten-dollar bill. A ten-dollar bill is the same as ten one-dollar bills (or two five-dollar bills).

1 2 3 4 5
6 7 8 9 10

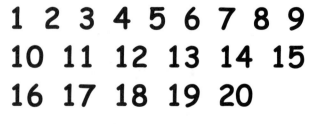

Twenty-dollar bill. A twenty-dollar bill is the same as twenty one-dollar bills (or four five-dollar bills or two ten-dollar bills).

1 2 3 4 5 6 7 8 9
10 11 12 13 14 15
16 17 18 19 20

5

SAFETY ISSUES

One of the most difficult aspects of parenting is keeping your child safe without being overprotective. Many children with autism lack a basic awareness of their own bodies, and this can lead to accidents. You can't prevent every accident, even if you follow your child around all the time. Still, you can always be aware of your child's relationship with her body, remaining vigilant around safety hazards. Your goal should be to prevent serious accidents without alarming your child and making her fearful.

Part Two includes a number of pages (pages 192–94) with safety images. These can improve your child's awareness of home and street hazards, but it is still essential to be aware of your child when you are out and about. She is not capable of exercising good judgment when it comes to traffic—she can't accurately assess the speed, or for that matter the intent, of an oncoming car. Besides, any distraction will take her mind off the fact that she needs to be cautious.

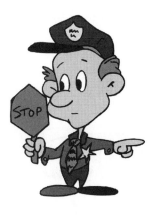

What Do You Say When They Ask, "Who Are You?"

It is very important for your child to be able to express who she is if she gets separated from you or another caregiver.

We have devised a few games to help you teach your child the name of the street you live on and the street number, as well as your names or the names of the people she lives with. The best way for your child to learn this information is through repetition. We urge you to play learning games until this information is memorized.

Making up a song is a fun way to help your child learn his address. For example, the following could be sung to the tune of "Mary Had a Little Lamb."

I live on Elm Street, Elm Street, Elm Street
I live on 1205 Elm Street
And my dad's name is Joe Smith.

Another way to reinforce learning the address is to write it on a piece of paper and have your child trace it with his hand as you say it out loud.

Play a game of memory with your child. On separate pieces of paper, write each one twice: the street numbers, the name of the street, the child's name, and the parents' names. Have your child turn the pieces over as a memory game, matching the numbers and names. Be sure to speak the words out. If you have devised a song, 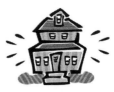 you can sing each item as its card is turned over. Match the pieces of paper. Then put them in order: the street number, then the name of the street and her name followed by your names.

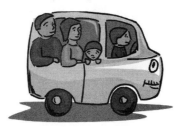

911

Knowing how to get help in an emergency is a complicated concept for a child to learn. But heaven forbid something should go wrong and your child's caregiver ends up unconscious on the floor or there's a fire in the house!

How do you teach your child to get help? As you know, many children on the autistic spectrum are uncomfortable talking on the telephone, so you need to help them overcome this fear. One way of doing this is to encourage short phone conversations with friends and family.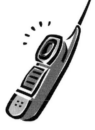

Teach your child how to dial 911. Break the process into small steps, making sure not to go to the next step until the previous one is mastered. Practice on an unplugged telephone. Let your child know that pushing the buttons 911 will bring help to your house. Show a picture of a police officer, paramedic and fire truck (they'll all probably come if he dials 911).

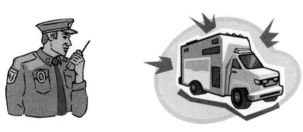

Have him master "dialing" 911 on the unplugged phone.

Teach him to say, "Help, my name is Mark and I need help." (You should decide for yourself whether to teach him to tell the dispatcher that he is autistic.)

Create visual aids to keep by the telephone:

FIRE

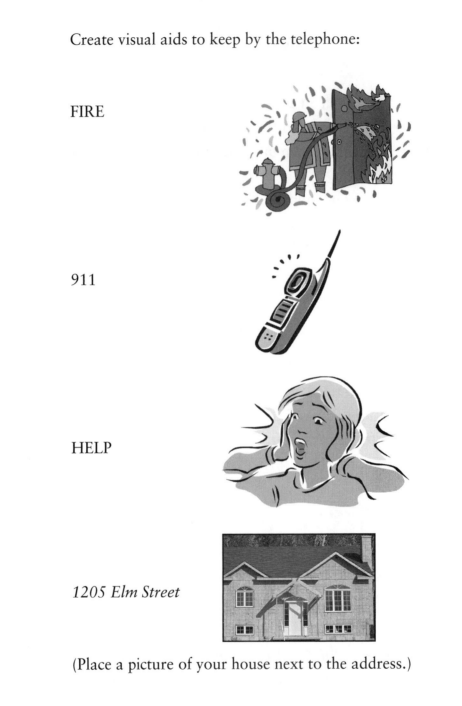

911

HELP

1205 Elm Street

(Place a picture of your house next to the address.)

The difficult part of this is teaching your child how to identify a true emergency. If your child decides to dial 911 because you are taking a nap, that will not go over well with you or the police.

6

PLAYING DETECTIVE WITH BEHAVIORAL PROBLEMS

When your child begins to act out, something is wrong. When he cried as an infant you had to determine the cause: hunger, wet diapers, an earache—you remember. Unfortunately, when a child on the autistic spectrum has difficulty expressing what's wrong, we have to resort to the same detective strategies we used when he was an infant to figure out what is causing his discomfort.

This chapter does not aim to provide a weighty treatise on uncovering the reasons for behavioral problems. What we can offer are a few clues to consider. Just what is causing Joe to flap, spin, rock, scream? In time you will probably be able to figure out what is going on because the responses will be associated with similar situations. Every time he wears a wool sweater Joe starts to rub his arms and pull at his clothes. It could be an allergy to wool, or perhaps he just doesn't like the feel of wool on his skin.

Behavioral problems don't develop out of thin air. There is a reason for them. One possibility to consider is that you pay attention to your child when she does something you don't want her to do. Is this just an attention-getting device? Or are there things going on inside her body or brain that need to be discovered in order to prevent or relieve her discomfort? In the long run, working with a therapist who is intimate with behavioral problems will help you understand your child's unique responses to the world. We're here to give you hints at the myriad possibilities.

Ain't Misbehavin'

When your child is acting "funny," be sure to consider the following:

MEDICAL CONDITIONS

Children with special needs are not exempt from other medical conditions. It is important for your child to have a complete physical evaluation to exclude other syndromes or illnesses that might account for ongoing behavioral difficulties. For example, if your child is tugging at her ears and screaming, it may not be an autistic spectrum behavioral problem. She may simply have an earache! The real reason your child doesn't follow your instructions time after time might in some cases be a hearing problem. Here is a list of disorders that may contribute to behavioral problems:

allergies

attention deficit disorder

anxiety attacks

chronic infections (tonsillitis, sinusitis, etc.)

dental problems

mood disorders (depression, obsessive compulsive disorder)

seizures

sleep disturbances

ENVIRONMENTAL ISSUES

Another clue to consider is the physical environment your child is in. Is there anything in the restaurant that would make him want to escape into his world of flapping? Think about how you feel when you walk into a cocktail party where you don't know anyone. Would you like to retreat to the corner of the room and hide? Maybe as you have grown older the noise from a Metallica rock concert would send you up the wall. (Maybe not?) Take a look around your environment and try to put yourself in your child's shoes. (Are his shoes too tight?) Think about what could be making him feel uneasy.

Too much stimulation of the senses. Are the lights too bright? Is there a background noise that is annoying your child? Does

A common mistake in working with your special needs child is using communication methods that are not basic enough. Use a variety of methods to teach.

something smell bad? Does the feel of the chair she is sitting in irritate her skin? Are there motions in the room that might be affecting her?

The actual space she is in. Is it too confining? Or the reverse—too large?

The people in the room. Are there people around him he doesn't know? Are there too many people near him? Is no one close enough to him to make him feel safe?

Clues: Is she giving you any clues that could help you determine whether the environment is causing her to act out? Hands over the ears may be an obvious response to too much noise; not wanting to be near a particular person might arise from a strong smell of cologne; ripping at his clothes could result from something as trivial as a tag on the back of the shirt irritating his sensitive skin; flapping and spinning might indicate a lack of stimulation to the brain—or too much stimulation.

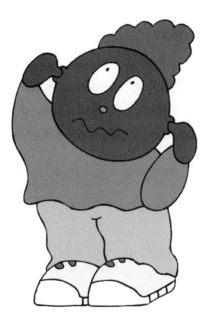

What's a Parent to Do?

So you're out in the world and your child is behaving in an inappropriate manner. What are you going to do? The first thing to do is remain calm and let go of any expectations that you might have had for the moment. This is only life happening and it will change. The next thing is to do your best to figure out why your child is acting out. Is it the environment? (See Ain't Misbehavin' on page 72 for suggestions.) If the environment is the cause, try changing it.

If your child is afraid, help her to calm down by giving her a full-body squeeze. Sometimes sensory input of this nature can be helpful to calm your child. Oftentimes your child might lose the sense of where her body begins and ends, or the stimulation is too great for her mind and senses to process. A squeeze has always been a great way for my son to shift his behavior, especially when accompanied with a tickle and a funny sound. Of course, try another tactic if this only heightens the anxiety.

You might also try handing your child a favorite toy. These transitional objects can be a very soothing force when your child is faced with stressful situations.

Getting the Behavior You Want

There are four basic reasons for behavior.

1. Escape from an environment or experience
2. Making a demand
3. Getting attention
4. Self-stimulation

When using behavior intervention to change behavior there are some basic things you need to know.

Don't reward negative behavior. If your child is displaying inappropriate behavior, do not bribe him with something to make him stop. This only encourages him to act that way again! We've all resorted to bribery at one time or another: "If you stop spitting, I'll give you a candy." It might work in the moment, but in the long run this will only encourage the inappropriate behavior.

Steps that lead to behavioral change:

1. Define your expectations.
   Make sure your desired behavior is understood before *the inappropriate behavior begins.*
2. Change the environment if it's not supportive.
3. Identify atypical behavior.
   Be specific about what the inappropriate behavior is.
4. Determine the *how, what, where, when* and, if possible, the *why* of the atypical behavior.
5. Define the new (desired) behavior for your child.
6. Choose an appropriate motivator for the replacement behavior. (See Cookies on page 76.)

You must be clear and concise in communicating what type of behavior you expect. You must also be clear as to what the consequences are if the bad behavior persists. (Don't threaten something you don't mean.) The basic tenet of behavior modification is to reward your child if she is giving you the behavior you are expecting. Reward positive behavior immediately!

What is **Behavior Intervention?** It is a method of using positive reinforcement and consequences to decrease inappropriate behaviors and increase communication, learning and appropriate social behaviors.

Motivators (Cookies)

Motivators are cookies or anything else that *motivates* your child. Reward positive behavior immediately with one of three types of motivators:

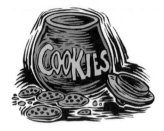

PRIMARY

Food, drink, warmth, comfort, etc.

Primary motivators are objects of need and desire—you will have to find out what these are for your child. These usually work best as a food treat (cookies, for example). The hope is to work up to secondary and then to intrinsic motivators.

SECONDARY

Checks, stickers, points, etc.

These tokens can be accumulated to gain special treats (toys, candy, etc.). The use of these items is called a token economy. You can set up a simple or elaborate menu of items or special events that can be purchased with accumulated tokens. We have included some tokens on page 217 that can be cut out and laminated. You and your child can also work together to make your own tokens. That way she can share in the experience of creating her own reward system.

INTRINSIC

Social attention, praise, pride in accomplishment, etc.

Because the child with autism is not as "connected" with the world as the typical child, these motivators often do not do as well. It is harder for the child with autism to enjoy and embrace the intrinsic reward offered. That is why Primary and Secondary rewards are much more effective in changing inappropriate behavior. The goal is that over time, as the child's relationship with the world is felt and defined, intrinsic reinforcers will be embraced more readily.

Positive Reinforcement Visuals

When you want to reinforce a given behavior, you can use positive reinforcement visuals. Any image can be used effectively if it is something that your child responds to and likes, such as trains, planes, rockets, flowers, dolls, horses, etc.

Select an image and break it down into pieces that can be put together as your child accomplishes the targeted behavior. For items that have faces or heads, make the head the first piece you give. That way you won't end up with a headless horse or doll. When the picture is completed, then your child receives whatever secondary reinforcement had been agreed upon at the beginning of the time frame.

You can also use words written on a picture as a means of acknowledging the targeted behavior instead of making a puzzle. For example, use a picture of a rocket. Each time your child displays the desired behavior, he gets another "stage" on the rocket. You can write on the rocket a word of praise or just the name of the rocket piece (Stage 1, Stage 2, Stage 3). When he has completed the rocket, he can blast off to his reward!

Make sure your child knows what the consequences for inappropriate behavior are. Be prepared to follow through with them.

Blast off!!!

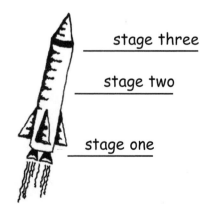

stage three

stage two

stage one

EXAMPLES OF
POSITIVE REINFORCEMENT VISUALS

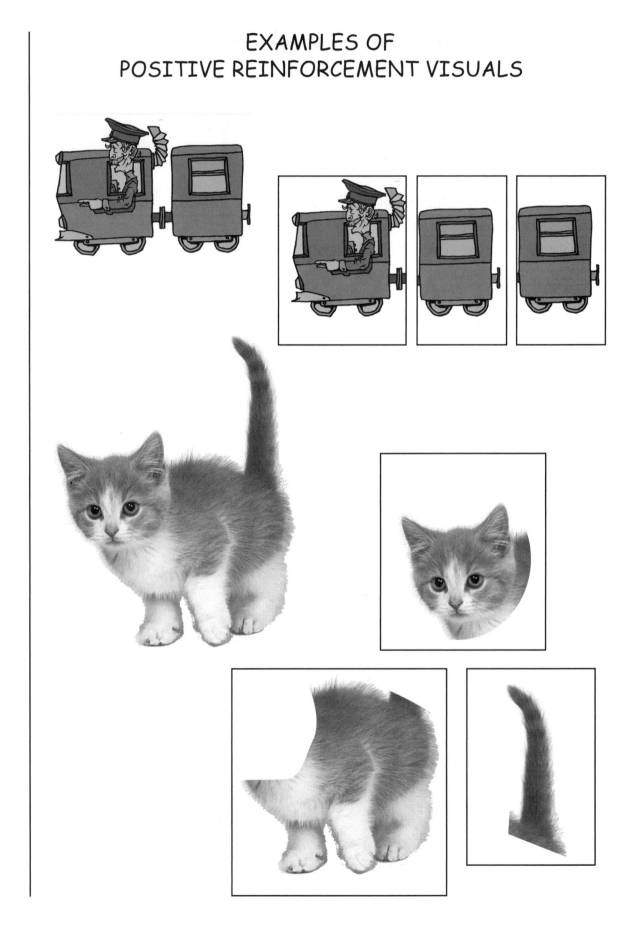

RESOURCES

Addresses of local autistic societies can be obtained from the Autism Society of America (ASA) headquarters in Maryland or from their website.

Autism Society of America
7910 Woodmont Avenue, Suite 300
Bethesda, MD 20814-3067
Phone: 301-657-0881 or 800-3AUTISM
Fax: 301-657-0869
www.autism-society.org; e-mail: info@autism-society.org

EARLY INTERVENTION

Every state is required to provide a free evaluation and early-intervention services for children. To find out whom to contact in your state, consult the **National Information Center for Children and Youth with Disabilities** (funded by the Department of Education) at 800-695-0285 or nichcy.org/index.html. Ask about support groups in your area as well.

RESOURCES ON THE WEB

Autism—PPD Resources Network
www.autism-pdd.net

Autism Research Institute - DAN
(Defeat Autism Now)
www.defeatautismnow.com

Autism Society of America
www.autism-society.org

Center for the Study of Autism
www.autism.org

Cure Autism Now
www.cureautismnow.org

Families for Early Autism Treatment
www.feat.org

MAAP Services for the Autism Spectrum
www.maapservices.org

National Alliance for Autism Research
www.naar.org

Yale Child Study Center—
   Developmental Disabilities Clinic and Research
www.autism.fm

Asperger Syndrome Coalition of the U.S.
www.asperger.org

Online Asperger Syndrome Information and Support
www.aspergersyndrome.org

Future Horizons
www.futurehorizons-autism.com

VOICES FROM THE OTHER SIDE

Reading first-hand accounts by people with autism provides a new perspective on how your child might be experiencing the world. You can find detailed reading lists on many autism websites, but here are two of my favorite books by people with autism:

Thinking in Pictures: And Other Reports from My Life with Autism by Temple Grandin
   This insightful autobiography can be ordered at most bookstores.

Beyond the Silence by Tito Rajarshi Mukhopadhyay
   Written by an Indian boy between the ages of eight and eleven, this incredible book of poems is available through the Cure Autism Now website:
   www.cureautismnow.org/tito/index.html

Jim Sinclair, an activist and writer with autism, has his own website. There you will find many eloquent essays, including my favorite, entitled "Don't Mourn for Us." Every time I read it I am moved by his wisdom. To read Jim's writings, go to:

web.syr.edu/~jisincla/

The following websites are generated by people with autism.

Autistics.org
www.autistics.org

Autism National Committee (AUTCOM!)
www.autcom.org

Autism Network International
www.ani.autistics.org

"Ooops...Wrong Planet! Syndrome"
www.isn.net/~jypsy

Know Your Lingo

Backward Chaining: Breaking a task down into steps, then teaching the steps backward, beginning with the last step. Not until each step is mastered do you teach the step that comes before. A wonderful example of backward chaining can be found at BBB Autism Online Support Network:

www.bbbautism.com/aba_shaping_and_chaining.htm

Behavior Intervention (Applied Behavior Analysis): A method of reinforcing desired behavior and ignoring or punishing unwanted behavior. It was developed by Dr. Ivor Lovaas to reduce inappropriate behavior and increase communication, learning, and appropriate social behavior in children with autism. For more information, visit these websites:

www.lovaas.com
www.nas.org.uk/nas/jsp/polopoly.jsp?d=108&a=3345
http://autism.about.com/cs/behavorialissues/a/lovaas.htm

Floortime Intervention: A technique developed by Dr. Stanley Greenspan that uses directed play to help facilitate breaking into the world of the child with autism. For more information check out these websites:

www.stanleygreenspan.com

www.coping.org/earlyin/ftpres

Mindblindness: An inability to "read minds" by attributing mental states to other people, such as thoughts, desires, knowledge and intentions. (This "mindreading" is a skill people must use constantly in order to communicate and interpret and predict others' actions.) Building on many years of research, Dr. Simon Baron-Cohen identified this impairment in people with autism in his book *Mindblindness: An Essay on Autism and Theory of Mind.* To learn more, visit:

www.autismresearchcentre.com/arc/staff_member.asp?id=33

Token Economy: A token economy is a system in which a child earns tokens for targeted (good) behaviors. Once a predetermined number of tokens has been collected, he can trade them for an item or activity that he desires. Read more about tokens at this website:

www.polyxo.com/visualsupport/tokeneconomies.html

Systematic Desensitization: A method for reducing anxiety. The things that cause anxiety are presented gradually, from the least anxiety-provoking to the most. This process is paired with relaxation and/or positive reinforcement. You can find more information at:

www.guidetopsychology.com/sysden.htm

PART TWO

✣

Your Child's Workbook

Paste your picture here.

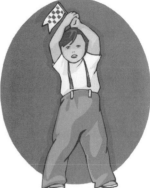

This part of my workbook is all about ME.

Follow the directions on each page.

All about Me
(Fill in the blanks)

I live in the house on _____ street.

The number of my house is_____.

My Mom's name is_____.

My Dad's name is_____.

I live with_____

_____.

Faces and Places

Paste a photograph
or picture of
your house here.

Paste a photograph
or picture of
your room here.

This is where I live.

This is my bedroom.

Paste a photograph
or picture of
your family here.

Paste a photograph
or picture of
your favorite place here.

This is my family.

This is my favorite place to visit.

Paste any photograph
or picture you like here.
It could be a picture
of your teacher, your pet
or someone you like.

This is a picture of

_____.

Paste a photograph
or picture of your favorite
vehicle here. (Is it a car, a
train, a bus or a plane?)

I like to ride in this.

Paste any photograph
or picture you like here.

This is

_____.

Paste a photograph
or picture of your favorite
toy or game here.

This is my favorite
toy or game.

My House

Draw a picture of your house.

I live at

_____

_____

_____

Write your street address here.

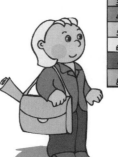
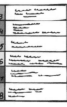

Schedules

Every day I have things to do. I keep a schedule so I know what to do next.

Cut out the pictures on pages 95, 97 and 99 and paste them into the spaces. Write what you will be doing on your schedule.

My Schedule

1. _____

Paste picture here

2. _____

Paste picture here

3. _____

Paste picture here

4. _____

Paste picture here

5. _____

Paste picture here

6. _____

Paste picture here

7. _____

Paste picture here

8. _____

Paste picture here

9. _____

Paste picture here

10. _____

Paste picture here

11. _____

Paste picture here

12. _____

Paste picture here

13. _____

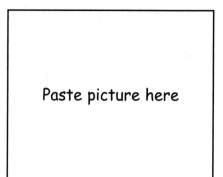

Paste picture here

14. _____

Paste picture here

15. _____

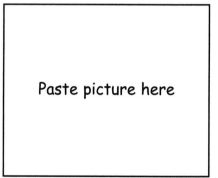

Paste picture here

16. _____

Paste picture here

Schedule Cutouts

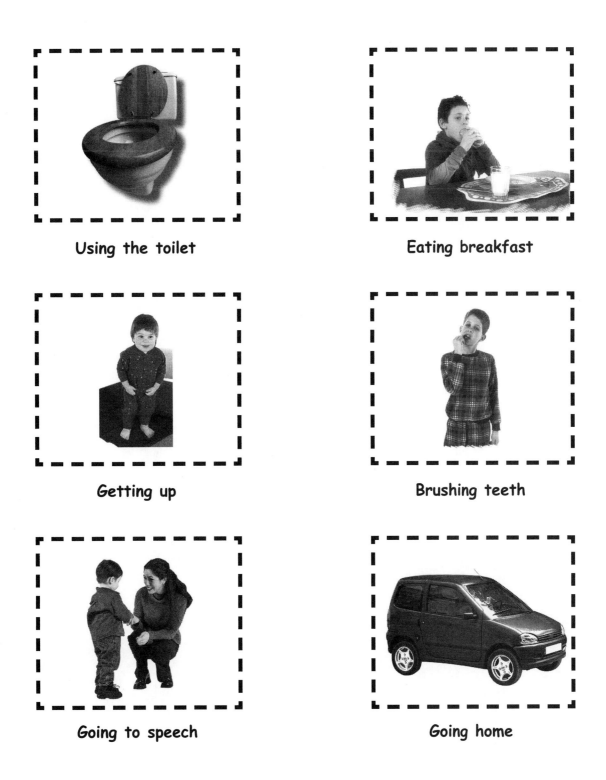

Using the toilet

Eating breakfast

Getting up

Brushing teeth

Going to speech

Going home

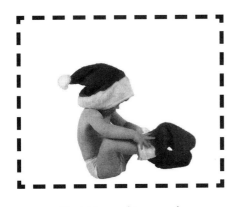

Getting dressed

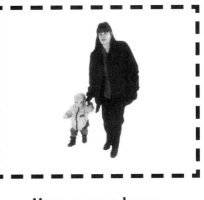

Mom comes home

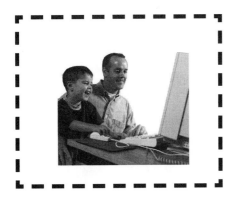

Computer time

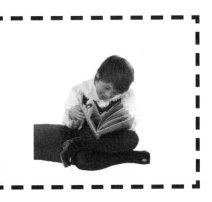

Reading a book

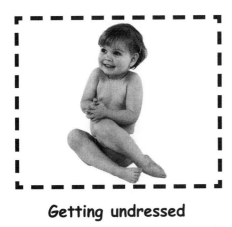

Getting undressed

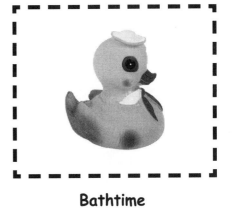

Bathtime

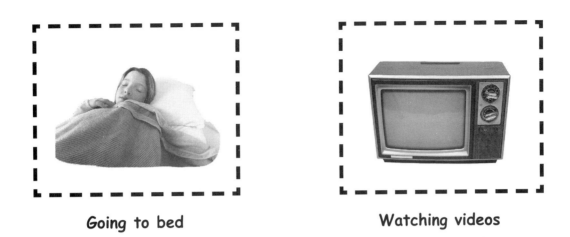

Going to bed

Watching videos

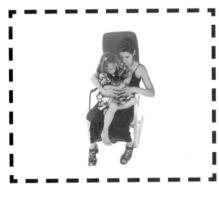

Rocking in chair

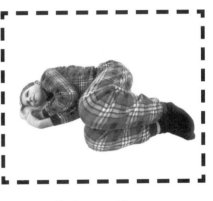

Pajama time

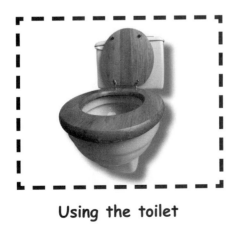

Using the toilet

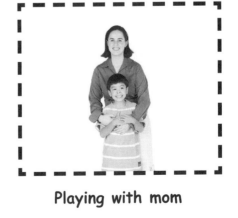

Playing with mom

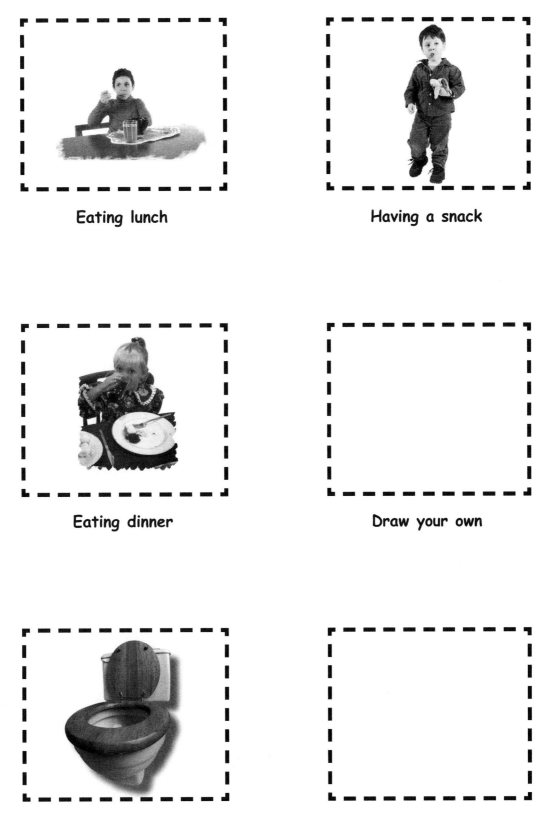

Eating lunch

Having a snack

Eating dinner

Draw your own

Using the toilet

Draw your own

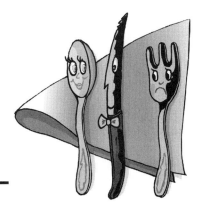

Setting the Table

Being part of the family means doing chores. Setting the table is a good way to help.

Follow the directions on each page.

SETTING THE TABLE

Let's learn the names of the utensils we use to eat with.

Here's a knife.

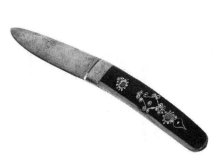

This is a fork.

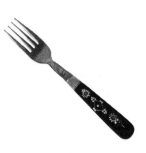

Here's a spoon.

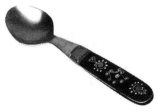

What else do we use on the table?

A glass.
What do we put in your glass?

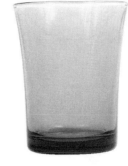

Napkins.
What do we use napkins for?

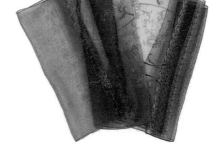

Here are the salt
and pepper shakers.

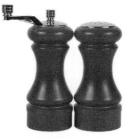

Draw a picture on this page and show where the knife, fork, spoon and napkin go on the table.

Now count how many people will be eating dinner tonight.

Paste pictures of where everyone sits. (Draw a picture of your table and chairs and paste pictures of the family members onto the chairs.)

What's Wacky?

The next two pages have a game to play. There are silly pictures to make you laugh.

Match the letter with the picture that shows how things should be.

What's Wacky?

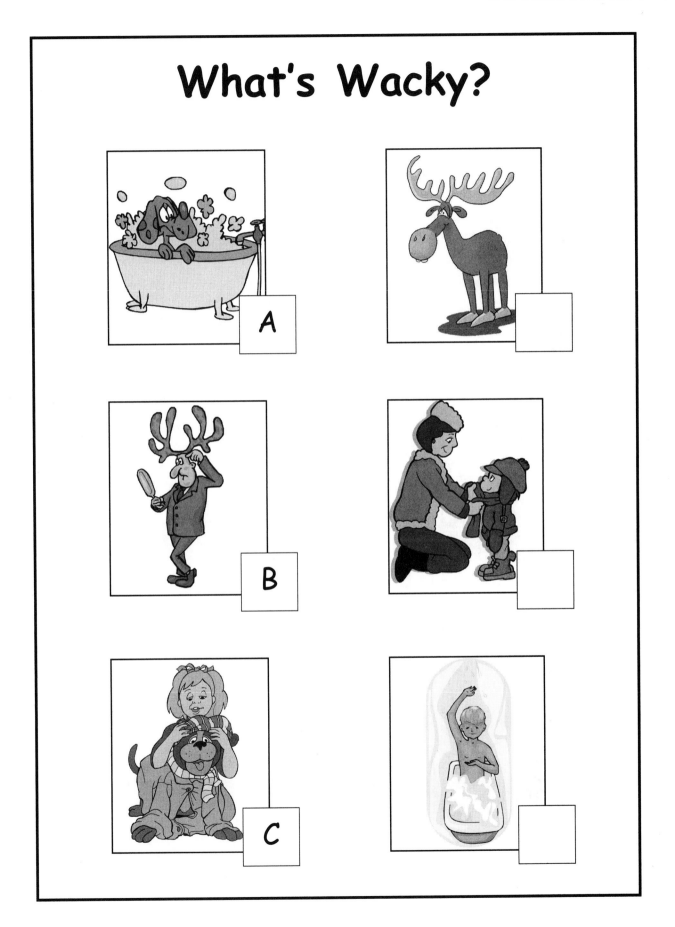

What's Wacky?

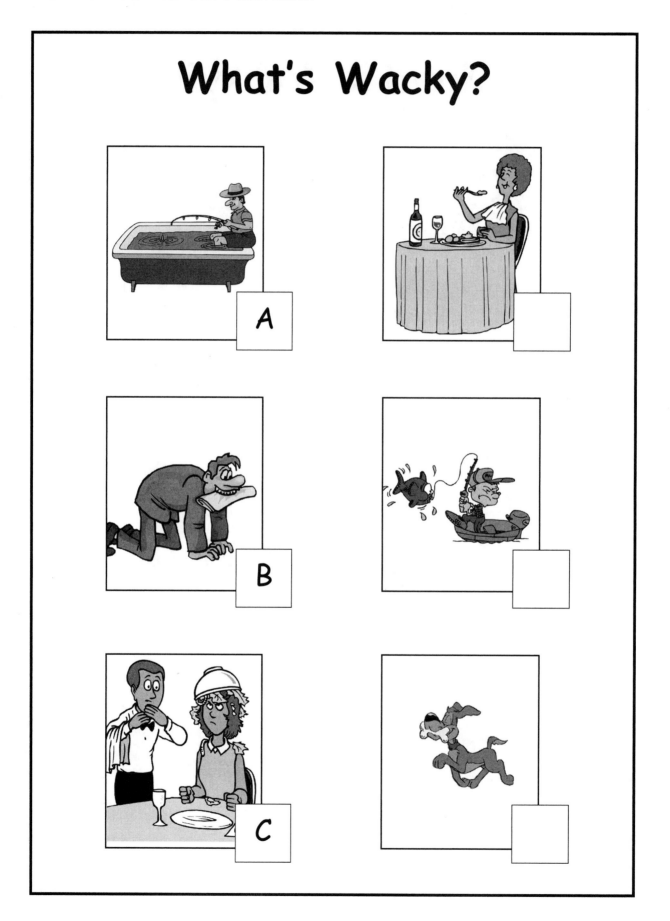

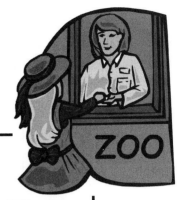

A Visit to the Zoo

The zoo is a place with lots of animals.

Find the pictures on pages 117 and 119 and paste them into the right boxes.

Lions make funny noises when they are hungry—they roar. Can you roar like a lion? (Roar for your child.)

Paste the picture of a lion here.
(Picture number 1)

Paste the picture of an elephant here.
(Picture number 2)

Elephants have long noses called trunks and they like to squirt themselves with water to keep cool.

Monkeys like to swing from trees and eat bananas. Do you like bananas?

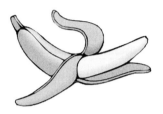

Paste the picture of a monkey here. (Picture number 3)

Paste the picture of a zebra here. (Picture number 4)

The giraffe has a very long neck. Sometimes he eats from the tops of trees.

The zebra looks like a white horse that has been painted with black stripes.

Paste the picture of a giraffe here. (Picture number 5)

The rhinoceros has two horns on his head, but he does not make music.

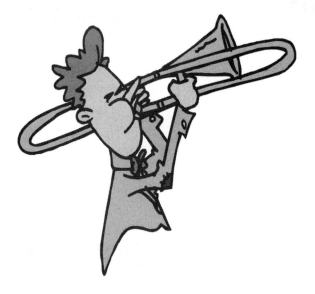

Paste the picture of a rhinoceros here. (Picture number 6)

Paste the picture of a gorilla here. (Picture number 7)

The gorilla walks on both her hands and her feet. Can you walk like a gorilla?

Bears like to eat fish and are very good at catching them. They also like to eat berries and grass.

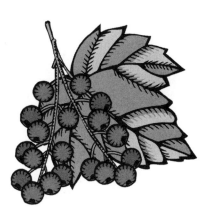

Paste the picture of a bear here. (Picture number 8)

Tigers have stripes. What other zoo animal has stripes?

Paste the picture of a tiger here. (Picture number 9)

ZOO ANIMALS TO CUT AND PASTE

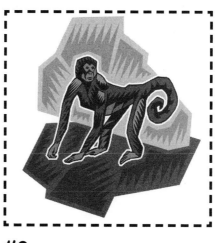

#3

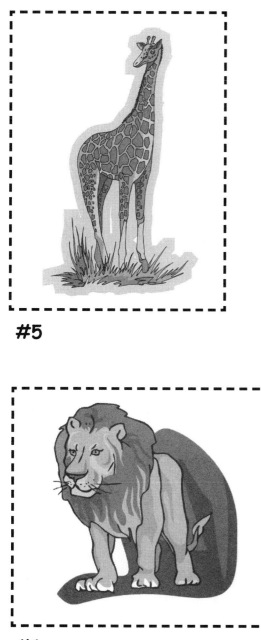

#5

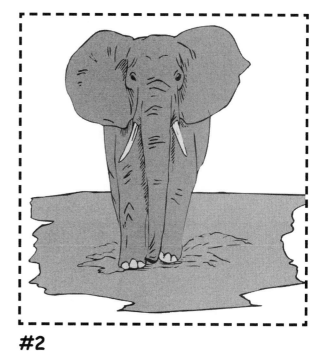

#2

#1

ZOO ANIMALS

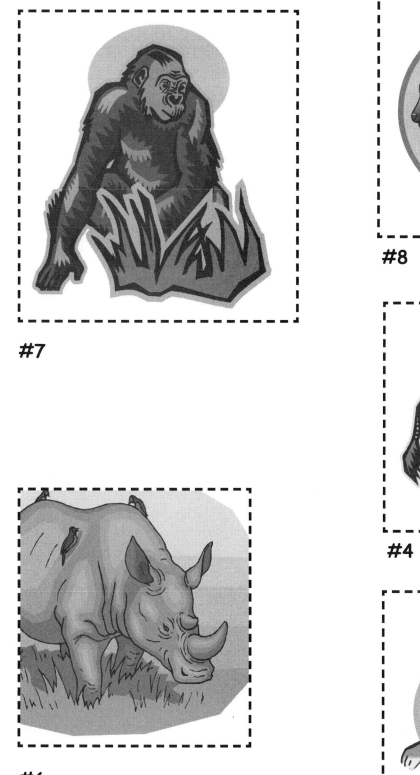

#7

#6

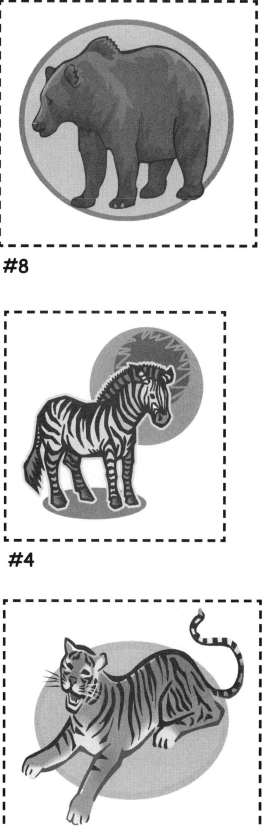

#8

#4

#9

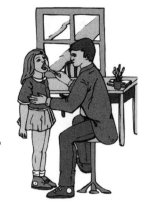

Visiting the Doctor

Look for the pictures that go with this story about going to the doctor's office.

Cut out the pictures on pages 129, 131 and 133 and paste them in your book.

The doctor is a person who takes care of me when I am sick and also gives me a checkup when I am well.

In this spot, paste the picture that shows the doctor checking the boy while his dad watches. (Picture number 1)

The nurse is the doctor's helper. The nurse usually weighs me and takes my temperature.

Paste the picture of a nurse here. (Picture number 2)

Sometimes you have to wait to see the doctor. Some children play games or read a book while they wait.

Some children like to sit by themselves.

Paste the picture of a boy sitting quietly here. (Picture number 4)

Paste the picture of kids playing a game here. (Picture number 3)

Paste the picture of a scale here. (Picture number 5)

When I go to the doctor I find out if I am growing. I stand on a scale and see how much I weigh. Some scales also have measuring sticks to see how tall I am.

The doctor has me lie down on a special table. The doctor lifts up my shirt to listen to my chest. If I feel funny, I think about something nice, like playing with a robot.

Paste the picture of a robot here. (Picture number 6)

Paste the picture of the examination table here. (Picture number 7)

Paste the picture of a doctor putting on gloves here. (Picture number 8)

Before the doctor and nurse touch me, they put on rubber gloves. The gloves sometimes feel funny when they touch my skin. It feels like touching a plastic doll.

The doctor looks in my mouth. The doctor uses a tongue depressor to push my tongue down to see the back of my throat.

I ask my mother to hold my hand because I don't like that feeling. The doctor makes me say "aaahhh."

Paste the picture of tongue depressors here. (Picture number 9)

In this spot, paste the picture of a boy opening his mouth so the doctor can look inside. (Picture number 10)

Paste the picture of the "ear flashlight" here. (Picture number 11)

The doctor looks in my ear with a little light. It is dark in my ear.

She also takes a little hammer and taps my knee. That makes my leg move by itself.

Paste the picture of the hammer here. (Picture number 12)

The doctor listens to my heart and lungs with a stethoscope. The doctor can hear my heart go "thump, thump, thump." Next time I go to the doctor I will ask to listen to my heart.

Paste the picture of a stethoscope here. (Picture number 13)

Paste the picture of a doctor listening with a stethoscope here. (Picture number 14)

My heart is also checked by a blood pressure cuff, something the doctor puts on my arm and pumps with air. It's like pumping air into a tire.

Paste the picture of the blood pressure cuff here. **(Picture number 15)**

A heart is a pump. It has a funny shape, not like the hearts you draw to say "I love you."

Paste the picture of a thermometer here. **(Picture number 16)**

When I'm not feeling well, the doctor checks how hot I am with a thermometer.

Sometimes I need to have a shot. The nurse or doctor sticks the needle in me. It makes me say "ouch," but it usually doesn't hurt very much.

Paste the picture
of a needle here.
(Picture number 17)

Paste the picture of holding
hands here.
(Picture number 18)

I like to hold my mother or father's hand when I get a shot. If I take five deep breaths I will be okay.

When the doctor's visit is over I get a reward. Sometimes I get an ice cream cone.

Paste the
picture of
an ice cream
cone here.
(Picture
number 19)

DOCTOR'S OFFICE CUTOUTS

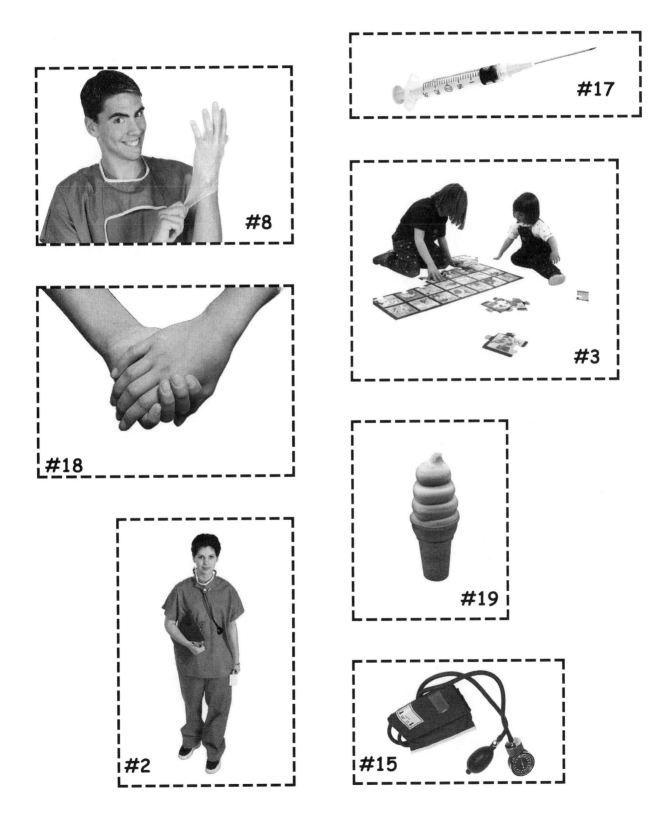

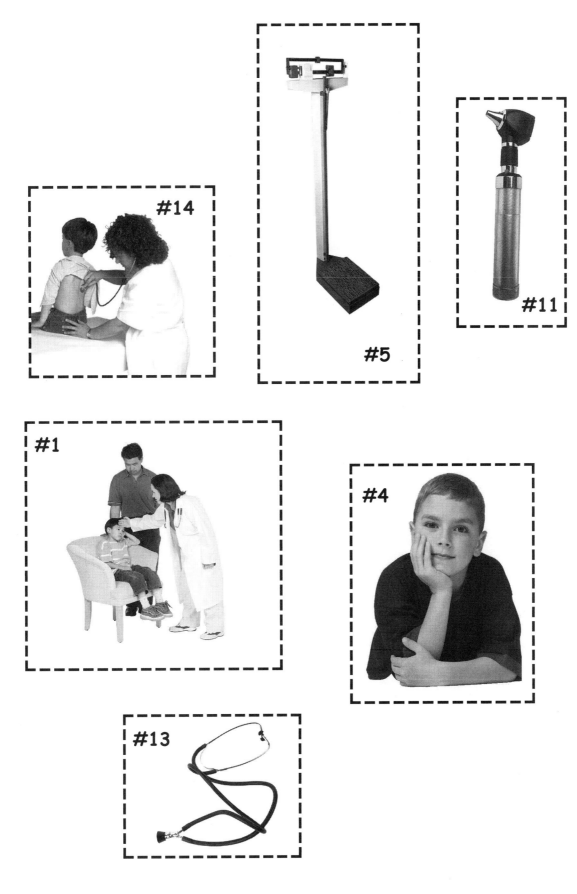

#14

#5

#11

#1

#4

#13

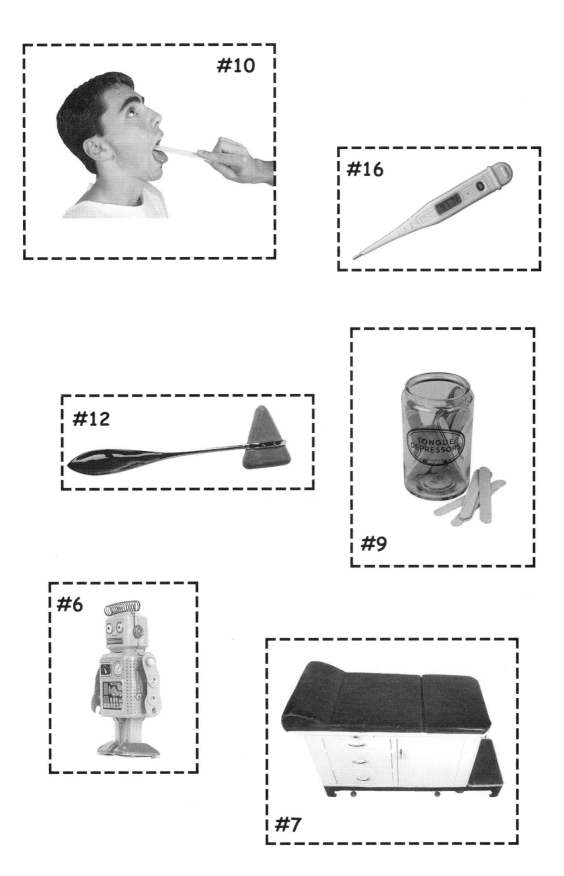

To Market, To Market

Here are some of the things that happen on a grocery shopping trip.

Cut out the pictures on pages 141, 143 and 145 and paste them in the spaces.

I like to go to the grocery store with Mom.

Paste the picture of a grocery list here. (Picture number 1)

Before we go to the store we make a list of all the things we need to get. Mommy lets me make one special choice to put on the list. Today I want cookies, so I put them on the list.

Paste the picture of cookies here. (Picture number 2)

Mommy always tells me when to get ready to go to the store. Sometimes she sets the timer to 10 minutes so I know when it is time to go.

Paste the picture of a timer here. (Picture number 3)

Paste the picture
of the car here.
(Picture number 4)

We drive the car
to the store. I put
on my seatbelt.

Paste the picture
of a boy wearing
a seatbelt here.
(Picture
number 5)

Paste the picture
of the grocery cart here.
(Picture number 6)

Mommy gets a
grocery cart
for us to put
the food in.

First we go to the place where the vegetables are and get the lettuce, broccoli and tomatoes that are on the list. Mom crosses them off the list.

Paste the picture of vegetables at the store here. (Picture number 7)

Paste the picture of broccoli here. (Picture number 8)

Paste the picture of bananas here. (Picture number 9)

Next we get fruit: apples, bananas and oranges.

Paste the picture of oranges here. (Picture number 10)

The list has "toilet paper" written on it. We go to the aisle with toilet paper. The rolls are soft and squishy.

Paste the picture of toilet paper here. (Picture number 11)

Paste the picture of the grocer stacking soup cans here. (Picture number 12)

Next we look for soup. We put the soup in the cart and then go to the cookie aisle.

Yay! We get the cookies and put them in the cart.

Paste the picture of the boy pushing a grocery cart here. (Picture number 13)

Paste the picture of the cashier
at the cash register here.
(Picture number 14)

Now we go to the
check-out stand.
The clerk takes
the groceries,
holds them over
the scanner and
puts them into
the grocery bag.

Paste the picture
of the bag of
groceries here.
(Picture number 15)

When I get home,
I get to eat my
cookie because I
paid attention and
helped Mom.

Paste the picture
of the boy
eating cookies
here.
(Picture
number 16)

GROCERY SHOPPING CUTOUTS

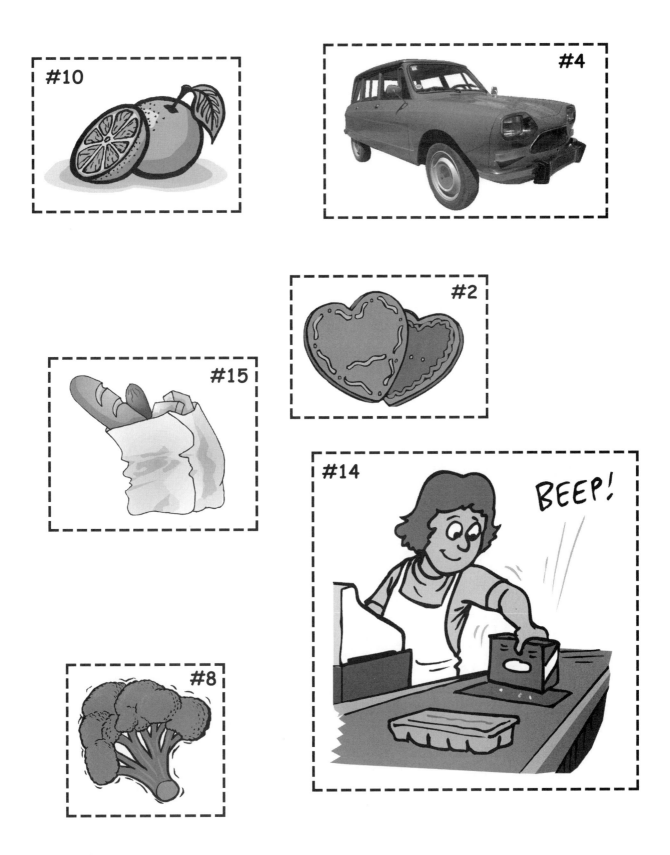

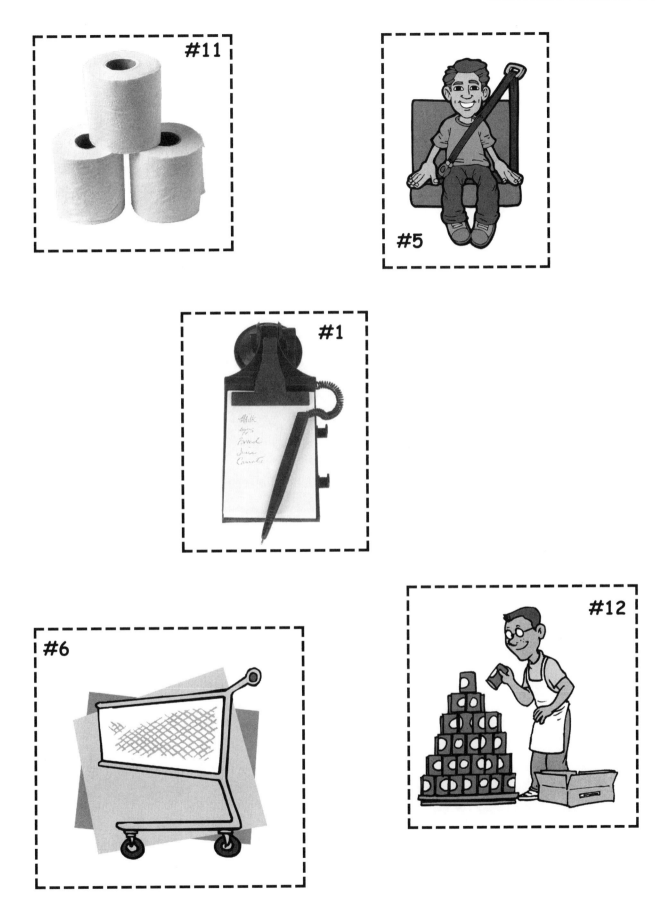

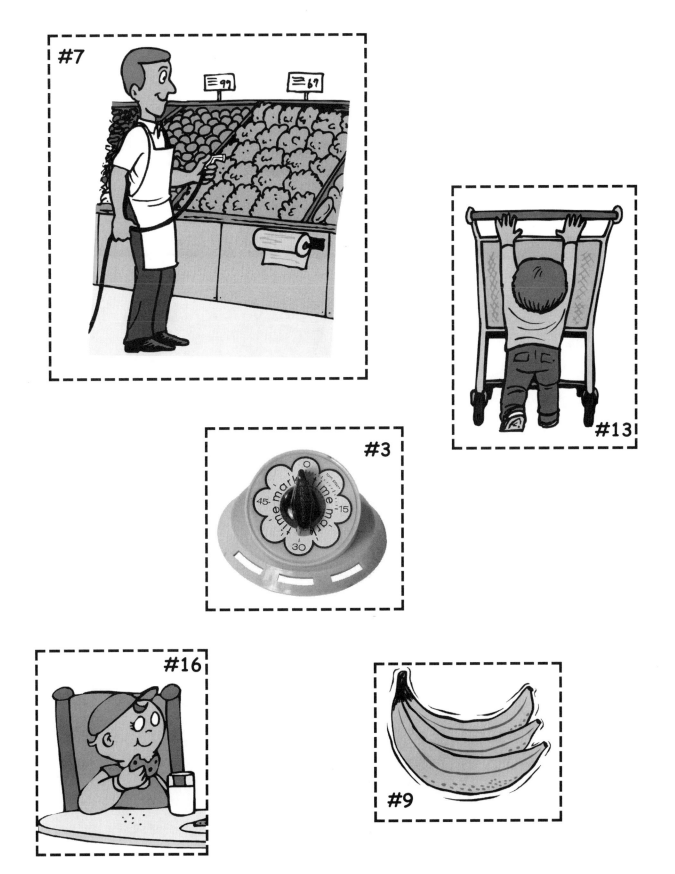

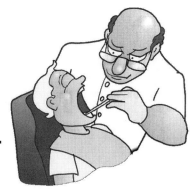

Going to the Dentist

Look for the pictures that go with this story about going to the dentist's office.

Cut the pictures out and paste them in your book.

I'm going to the dentist. The dentist is a person who takes care of my teeth. She also has a helper.

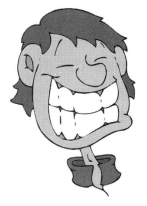

> Paste the picture of a dentist and hygienist here.
> (Picture number 1)

> Paste the picture of the teeth here. (Picture number 2)

The dentist has funny teeth on her shelf so that I can see how they look.

**Paste the picture of
the dentist's chair here.
(Picture number 3)**

When I go to the dentist I sit in a special chair. I can pretend I am flying in space.

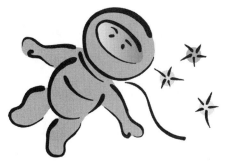

**In this spot, paste the picture of a girl opening her mouth to let the dentist work.
(Picture number 4)**

The dentist likes to have me open my mouth so he can poke my teeth to make sure they are clean and healthy. I close my eyes and pretend I am somewhere else.

Paste the picture of dentists' tools here. (Picture number 5)

The dentist has tools to clean my teeth and make them sparkle.

Sometimes I have to have a shot so that my mouth won't hurt. It makes my mouth feel funny.

Paste the picture of a needle here. (Picture number 6)

Paste the picture of a toothbrush here. (Picture number 7)

Then I get to go home. When I clean my teeth at home I use my toothbrush.

DENTIST'S OFFICE CUTOUTS

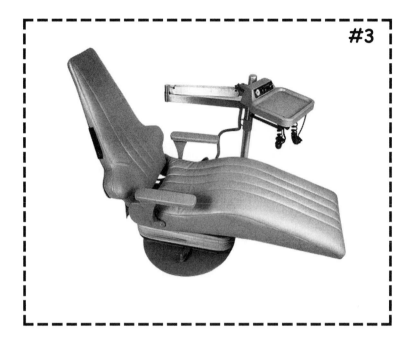

#3

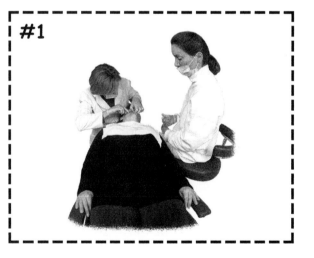

#1

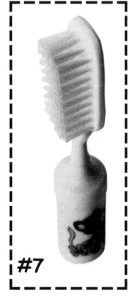

#7

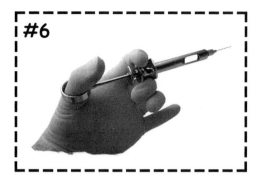

#6

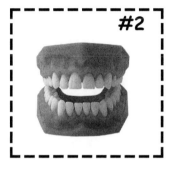

#2

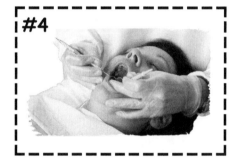

#4

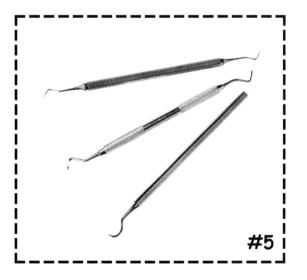

#5

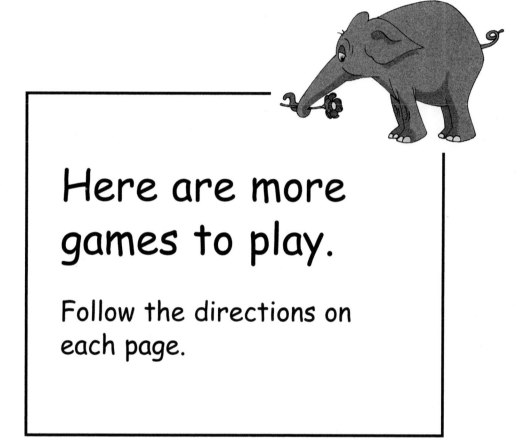

Here are more games to play.

Follow the directions on each page.

Getting Dressed
Matching Game

Draw a line from the clothing to the part of the body it belongs on.

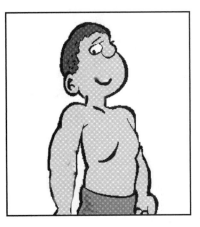 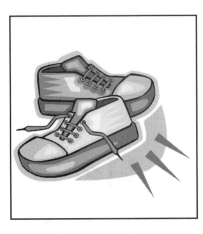

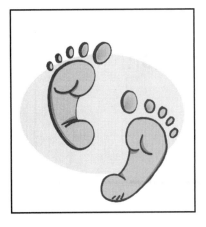 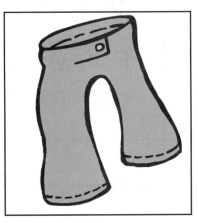

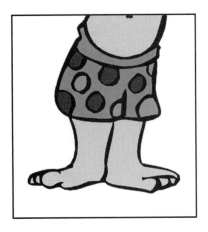 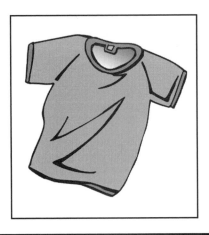

What I Wear Game

Which piece of clothing do you put on first? Which do you put on last? Cut out the pictures and put them in the right order.

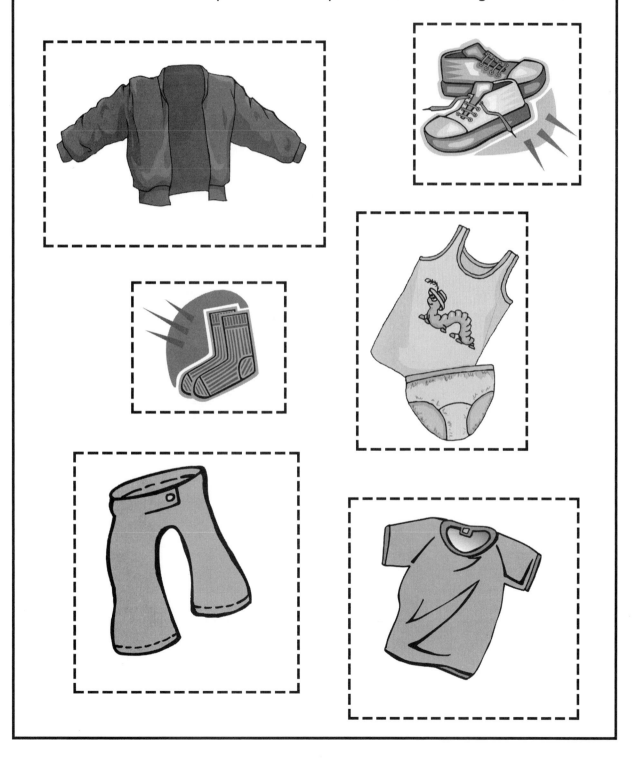

Rhyming

Some of these pictures have names that sound the same. Say the name of each picture. Draw a line between the pictures with names that rhyme.

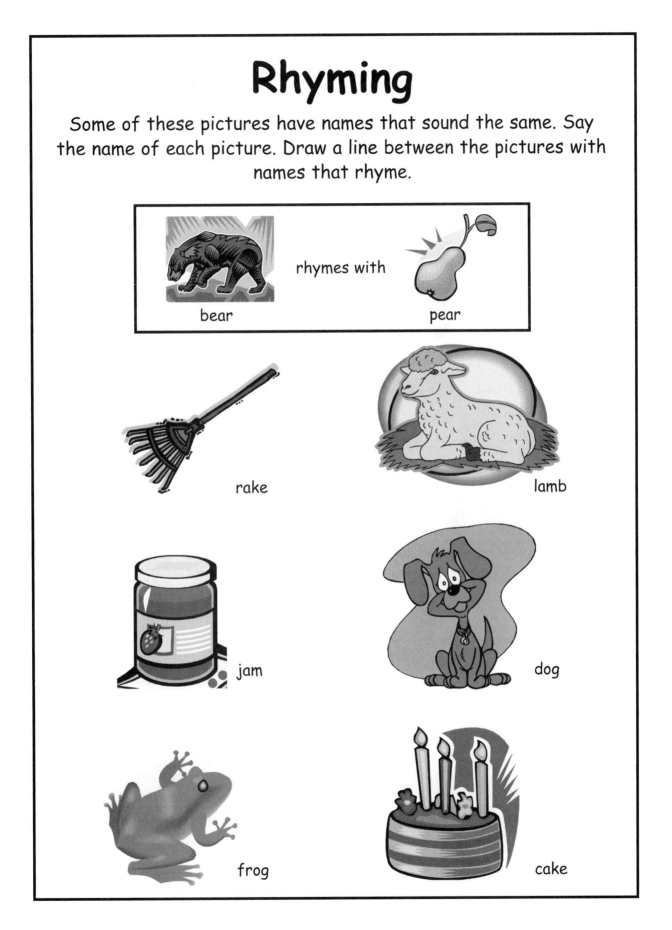

bear rhymes with pear

rake

lamb

jam

dog

frog

cake

Opposites

In this game, match the pictures that are opposites—NOT alike.
Draw a line between large and small, hot and cold, empty and full.

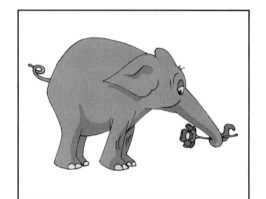

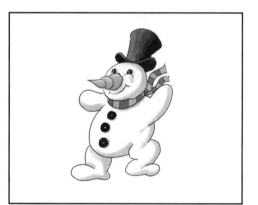

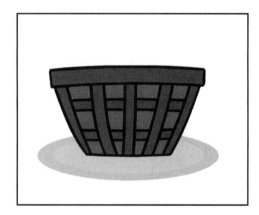

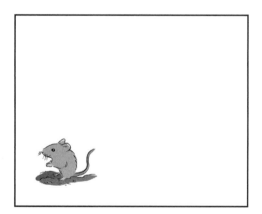

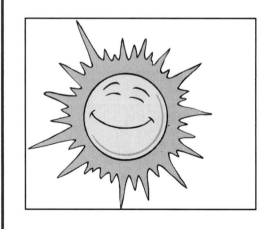

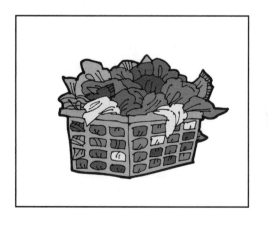

Which Comes First?

Write 1 in the square to show what happened first.
Write 2 in the square to show what happened next.
Write 3 in the square to show what happened last.

Making lemonade

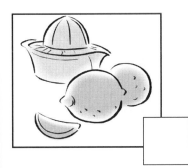

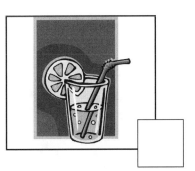

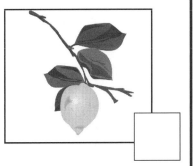

Birthday party

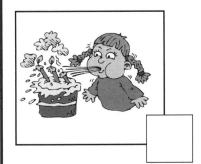

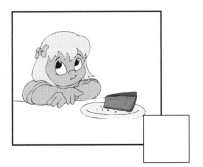

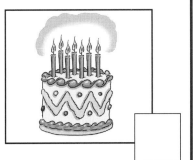

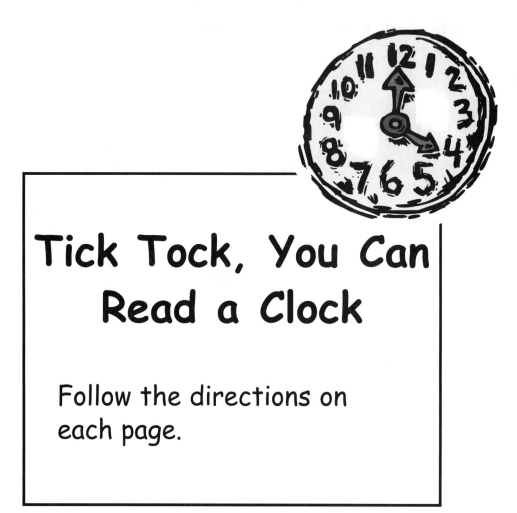

Tick Tock, You Can Read a Clock

Follow the directions on each page.

Parts of a Clock

Clocks have two hands. They are not like hands on your arms. They usually look like arrows. Here are two hands from a clock. One is called the BIG hand, and it shows you what the minute is. One is called the SMALL hand, and it shows you what the hour is.

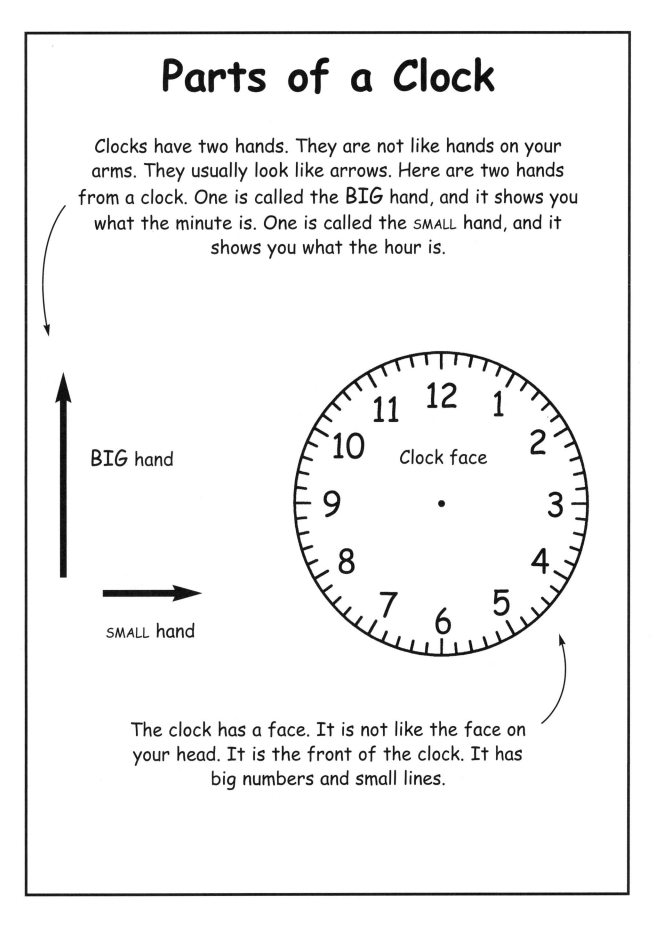

BIG hand

SMALL hand

Clock face

The clock has a face. It is not like the face on your head. It is the front of the clock. It has big numbers and small lines.

Clock Numbers

The numbers on a clock tell what hour it is. When the small hand points to a number, that number is the hour.

The numbers also mark time in five-minute sections. Look on page 166 and practice counting by fives.

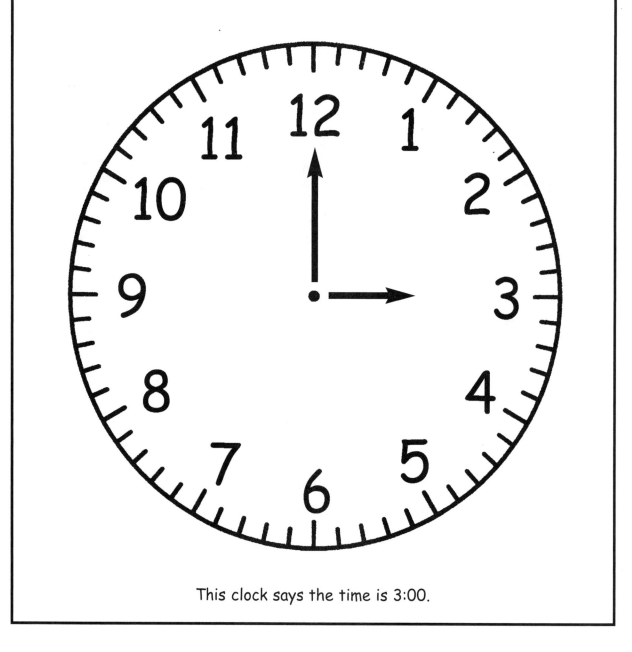

This clock says the time is 3:00.

Write the numbers that belong in the spaces below.

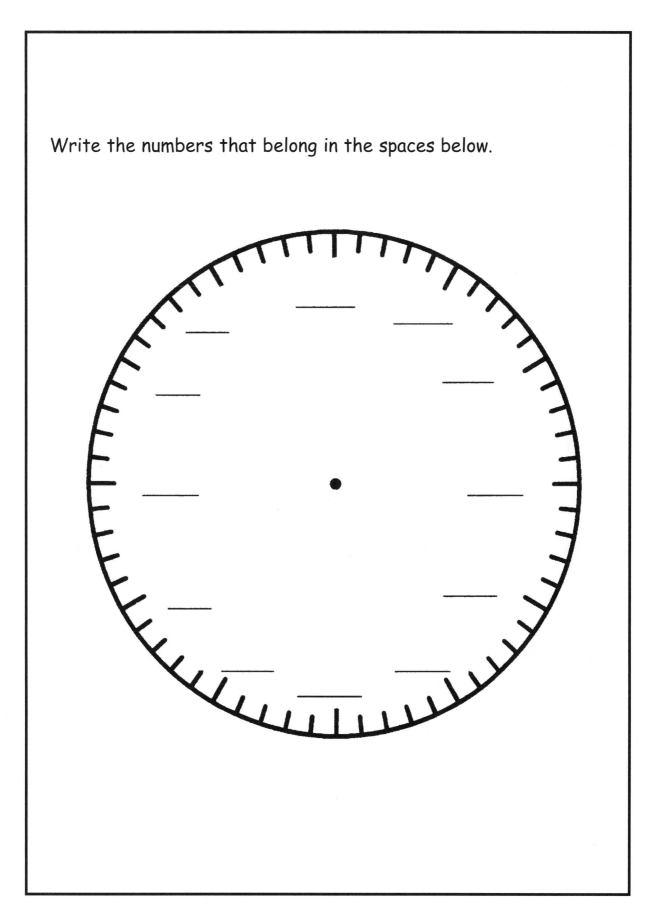

Number Grid

There are 60 minutes in each hour. Learn to count by fives to 60. Say out loud the numbers in the gray boxes.

1	2	3	4	5	6	7	8
9	10	11	12	13	14	15	16
17	18	19	20	21	22	23	24
25	26	27	28	29	30	31	32
33	34	35	36	37	38	39	40
41	42	43	44	45	46	47	48
49	50	51	52	53	54	55	56
57	58	59	60				

Count by Fives around the Clock

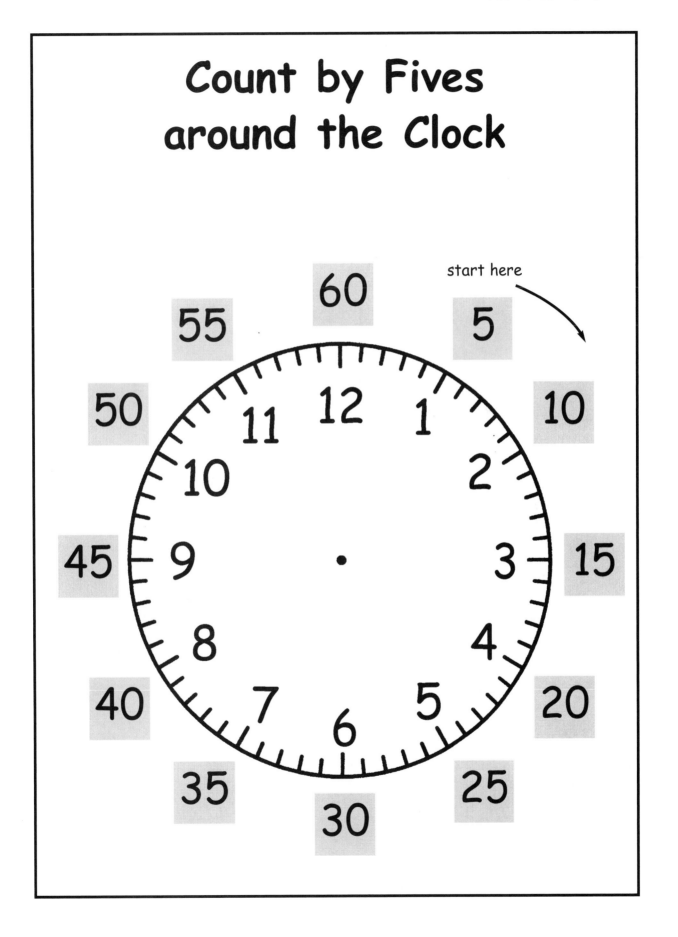

Draw the hands on clock **B** so that the time on the clock is the same time as clock **A**.

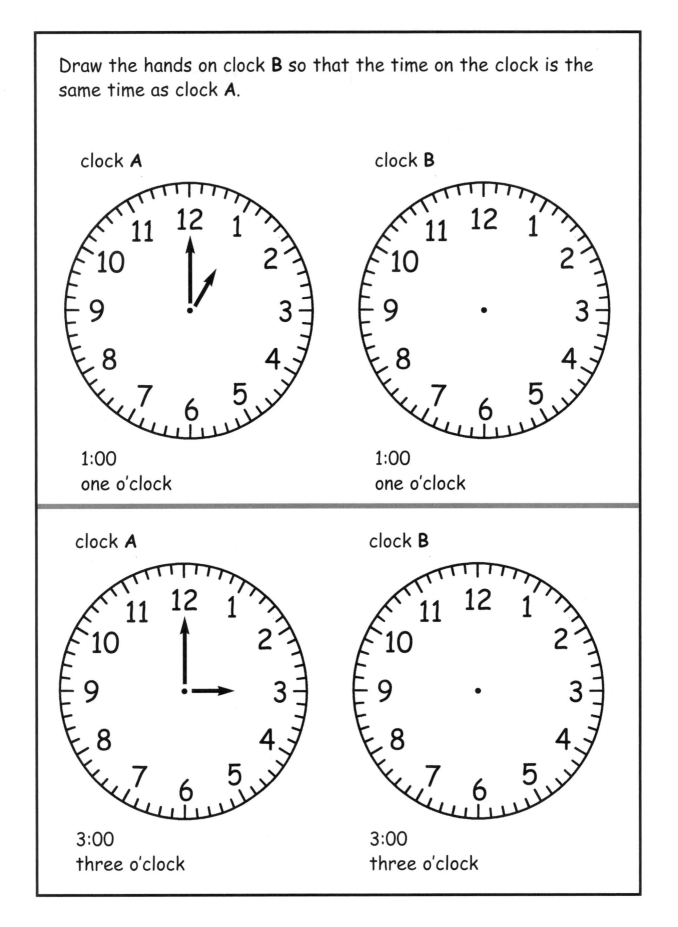

clock **A**

1:00
one o'clock

clock **B**

1:00
one o'clock

clock **A**

3:00
three o'clock

clock **B**

3:00
three o'clock

What time is it? Write your answer on the line below.

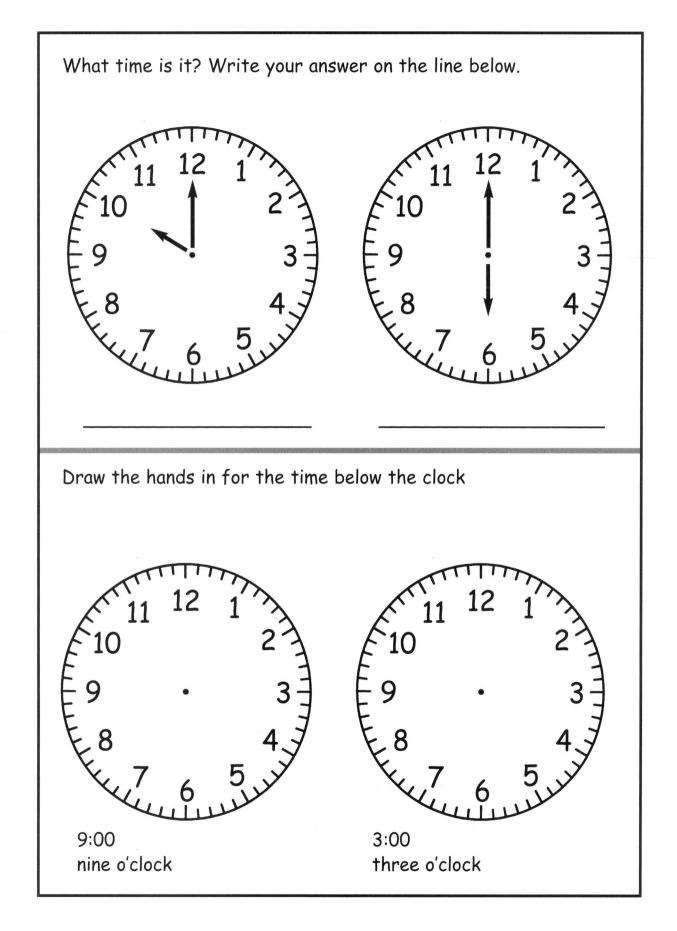

_____   _____

Draw the hands in for the time below the clock

9:00
nine o'clock

3:00
three o'clock

Three in a Row Bingo

Here is a game to play about your day.

Cut out the pictures on pages 173, 175 and 177. Pick cards from the stack and put them in a square that matches the picture. When you have three in a row, you will be able to say "Hooray, I did **Three in a Row** today."

Or

There are two copies of each picture. You can spread out all the cards and turn them face down. Play a game of memory by picking two cards at a time looking for a match.

What I Did Today— Three in a Row Bingo

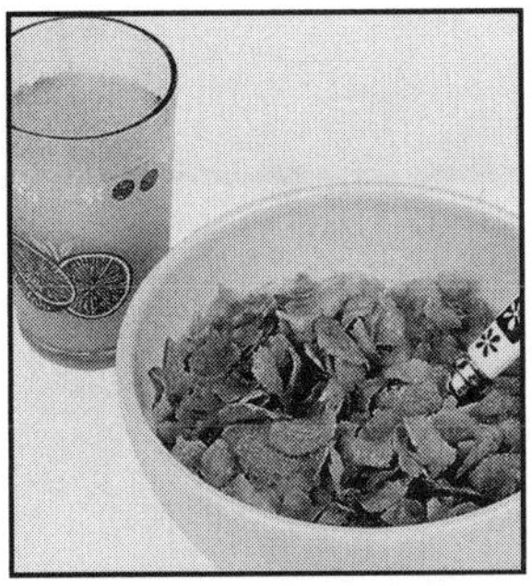

ate breakfast

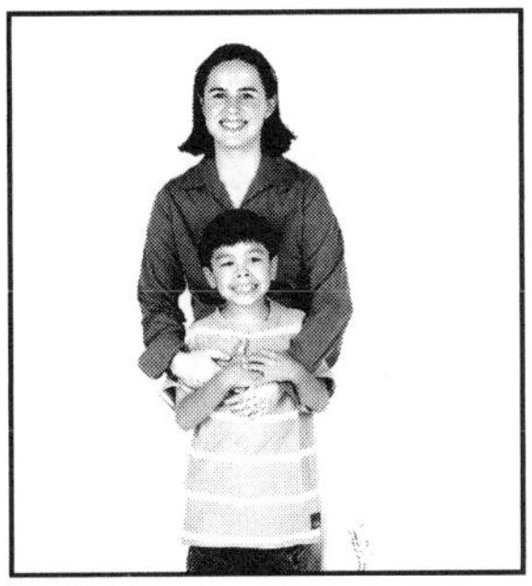

mom came home

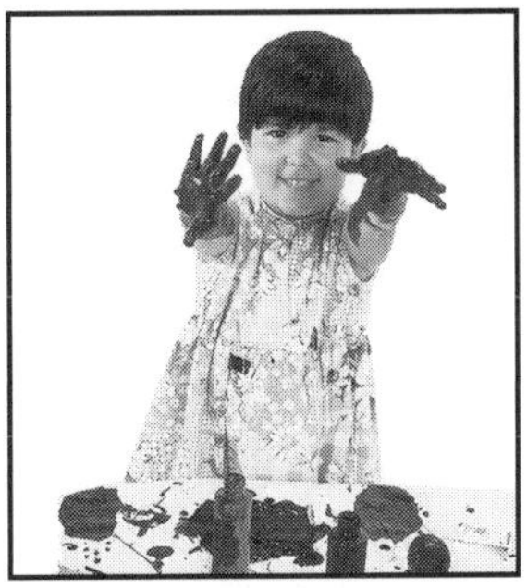

fingerpainted

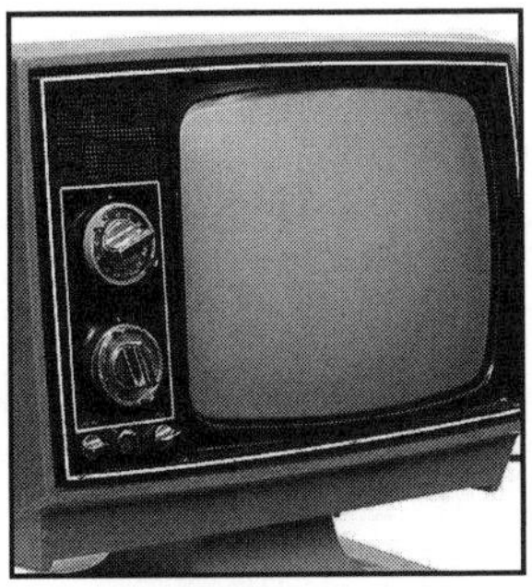

watched videos

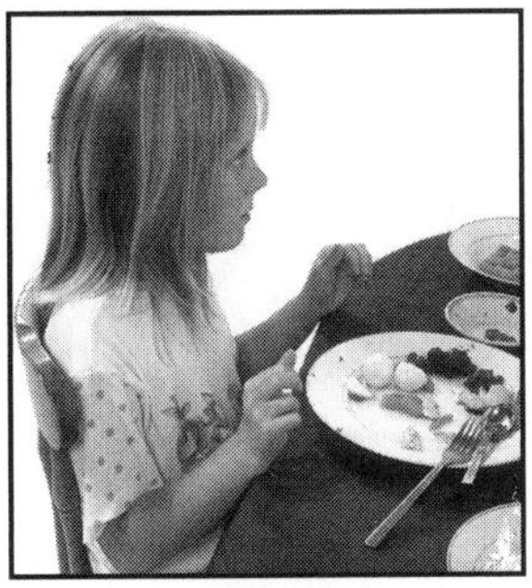

ate dinner

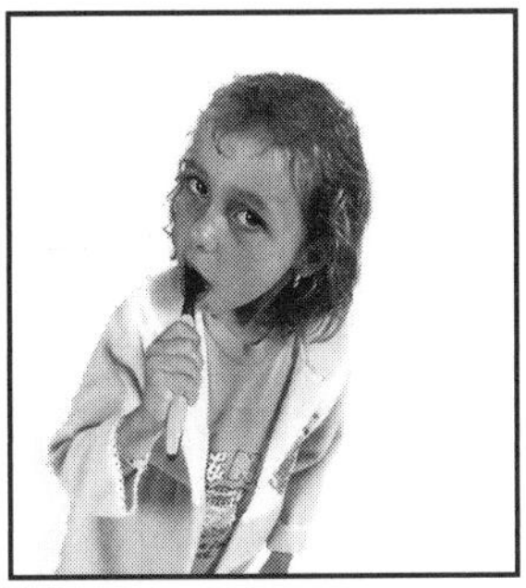

brushed teeth

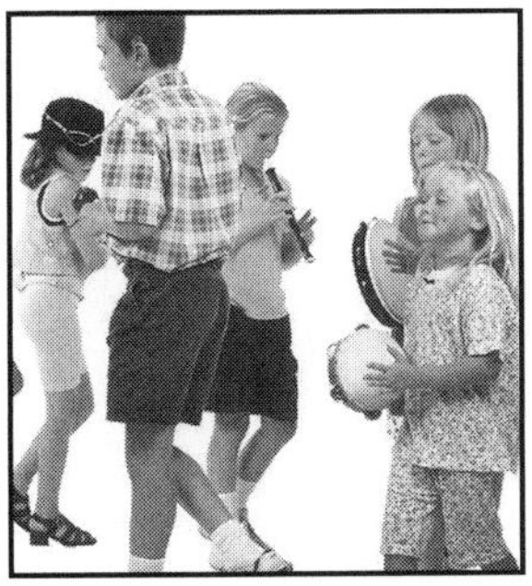

went to school

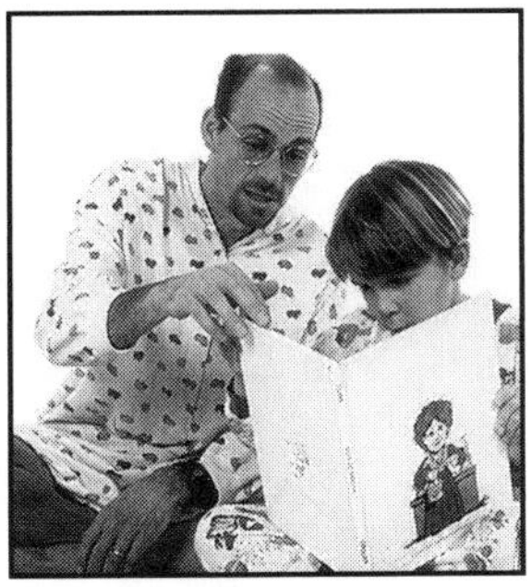

read story

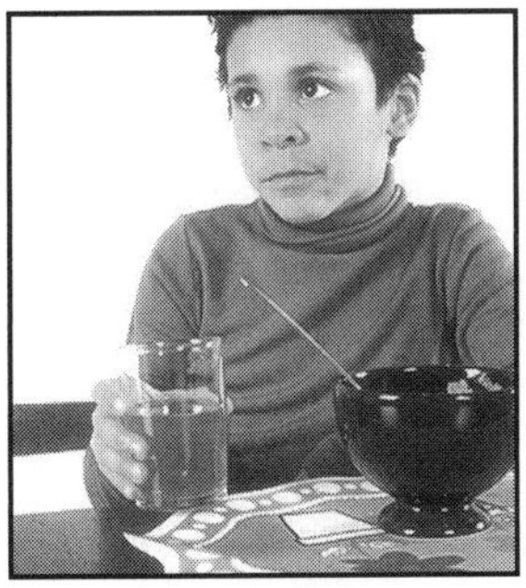

ate lunch

Three in a Row

Pictures to cut out

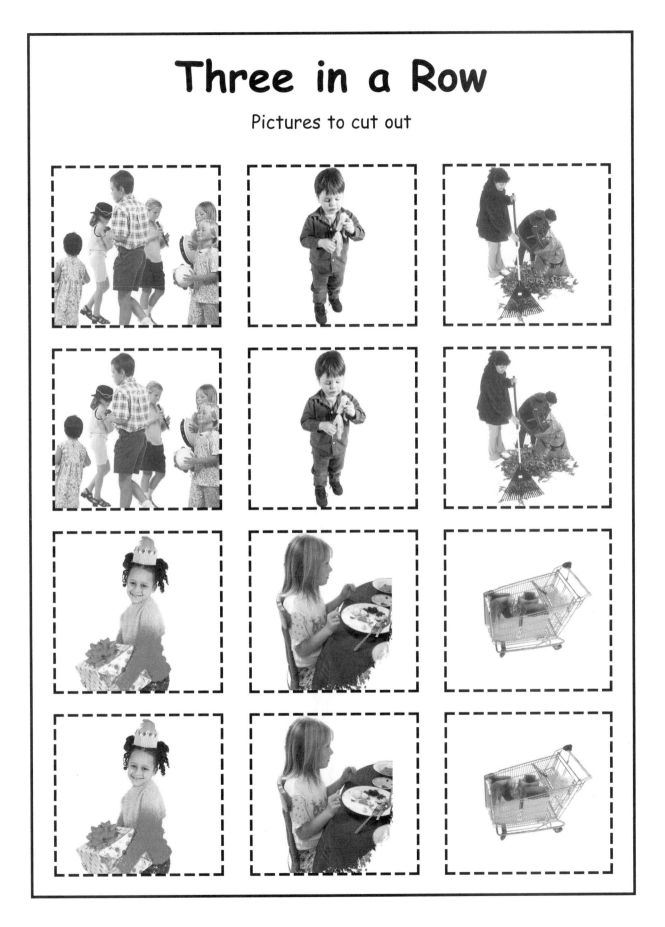

Three in a Row

Pictures to cut out

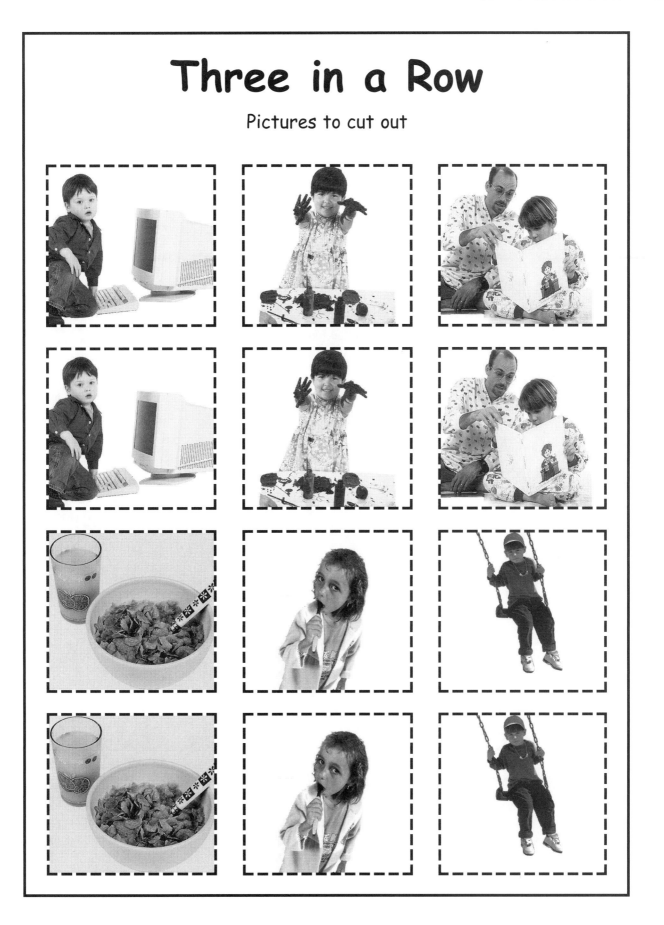

Three in a Row

Pictures to cut out

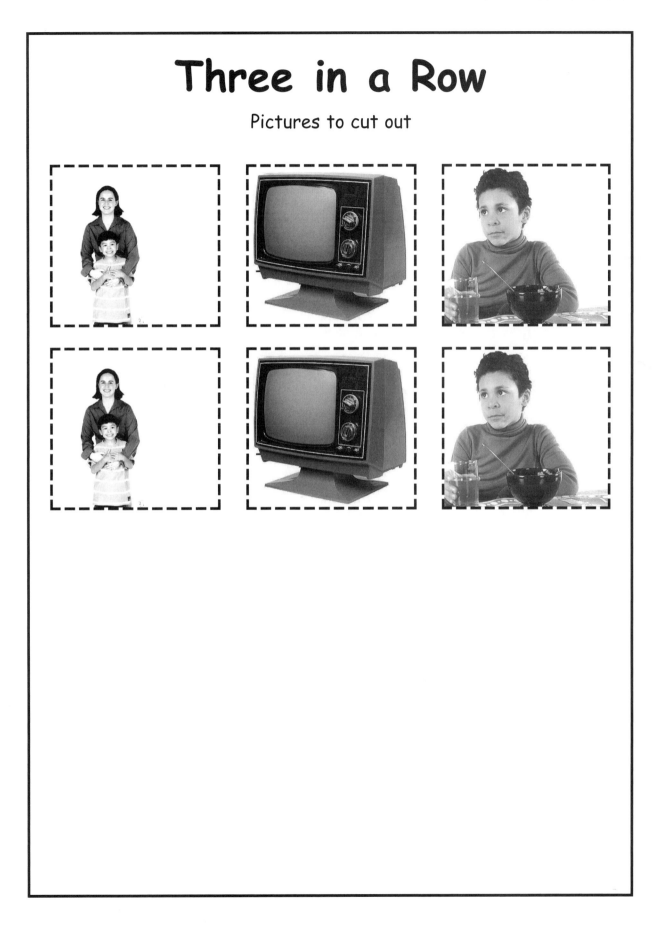

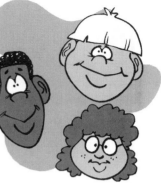

Reading Faces

Match the grown-up faces with the children's faces.

Can you find:

- two people who are sad?
- two people who are excited?
- two people who are mad?
- two people who are silly?
- two people who are tired?

Match each picture of a grown-up with the picture of the child who feels the same way. Write the picture's letter in the box.

Reading Faces

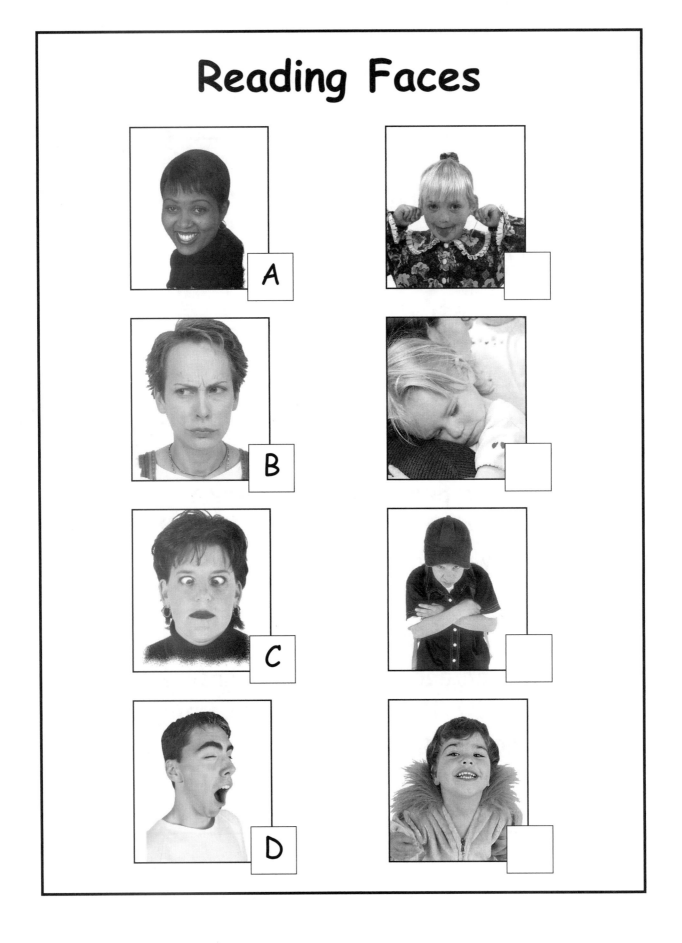

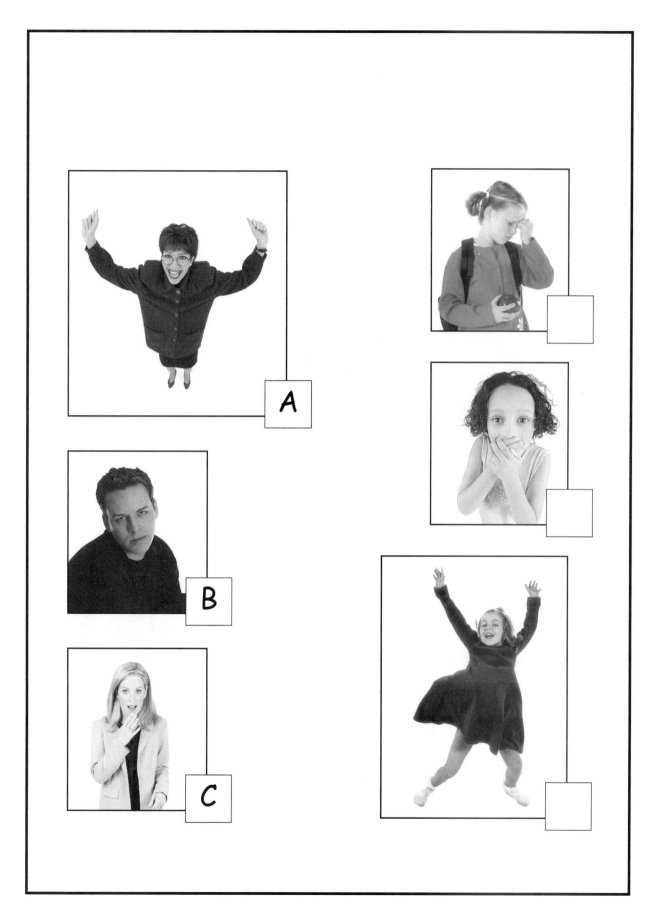

I am feeling...

Point to the picture that describes how you are feeling.

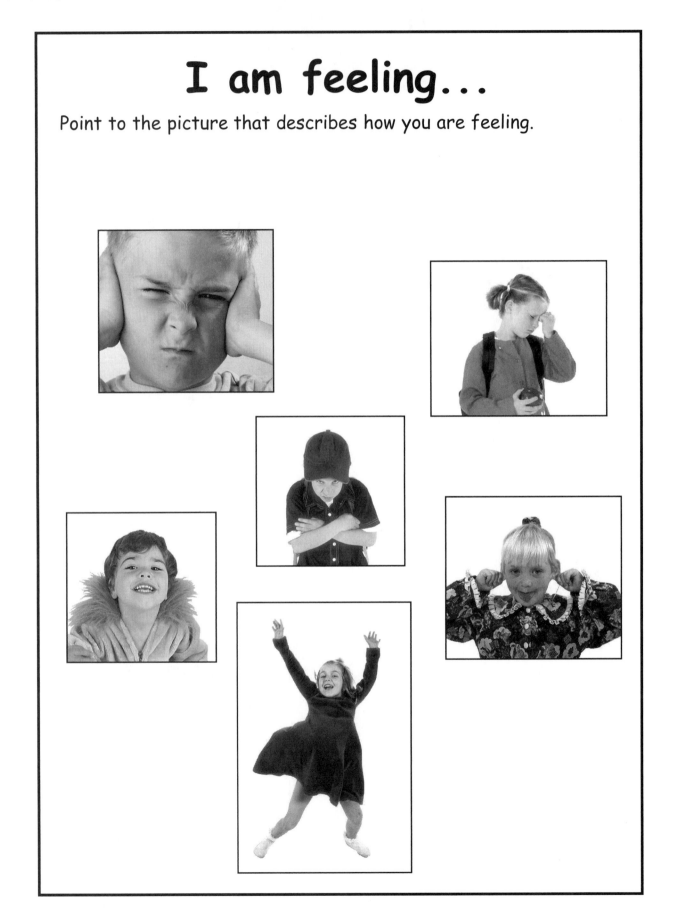

Money

It's important to know about money. Here are pages that help you learn your coins and bills.

Follow the directions on each page.

Learn Your Coins

When you go into the store you need money to buy things. Sometimes you pay with coins. Let's learn our coins.

One penny. A penny is brown.
You need lots of pennies to buy something.
1 cent

1

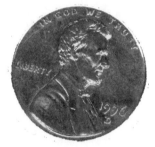

One nickel.
A nickel is silver.
It is the fattest coin.
5 cents

1 2 3 4 5

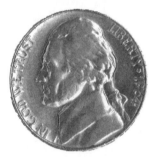

One dime. A dime is the smallest silver coin.
10 cents

**1 2 3 4 5
6 7 8 9 10**

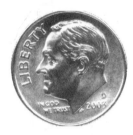

One quarter. A quarter is silver and bigger than a nickel.
25 cents

**1 2 3 4 5 6 7 8 9
10 11 12 13 14 15
16 17 18 19 20 21
22 23 24 25**

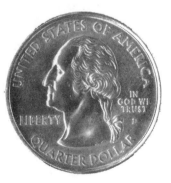

Coin Values

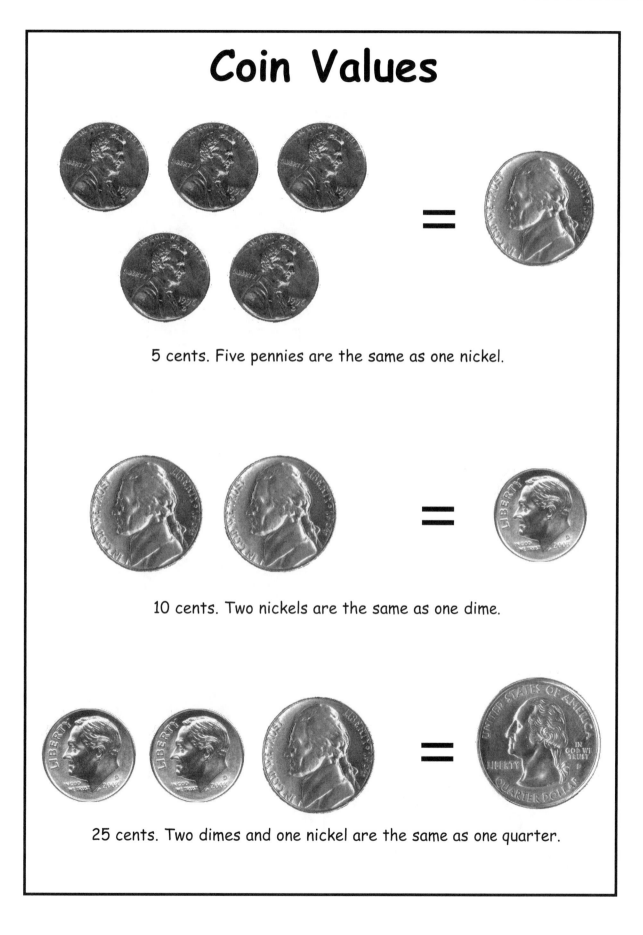

5 cents. Five pennies are the same as one nickel.

10 cents. Two nickels are the same as one dime.

25 cents. Two dimes and one nickel are the same as one quarter.

Paper Money

When you go into the store you need money to buy things. You pay with coins some of the time, but you will use paper money for most things. Paper money is called "bills." Let's learn our bills.

One-dollar bill. Dollars are used a lot.

1

Five-dollar bill. A five-dollar bill is the same as five one-dollar bills.

1 2 3 4 5

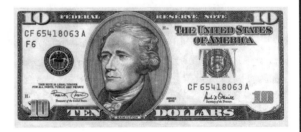

Ten-dollar bill. A ten-dollar bill is the same as ten one-dollar bills (or two five-dollar bills).

1 2 3 4 5
6 7 8 9 10

Twenty-dollar bill. A twenty-dollar bill is the same as twenty one-dollar bills (or four five-dollar bills or two ten-dollar bills).

1 2 3 4 5 6 7 8
9 10 11 12 13 14
15 16 17 18 19 20

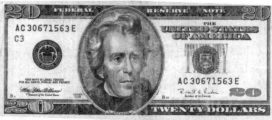

Coin Matching

Draw a line from the coins to their names.

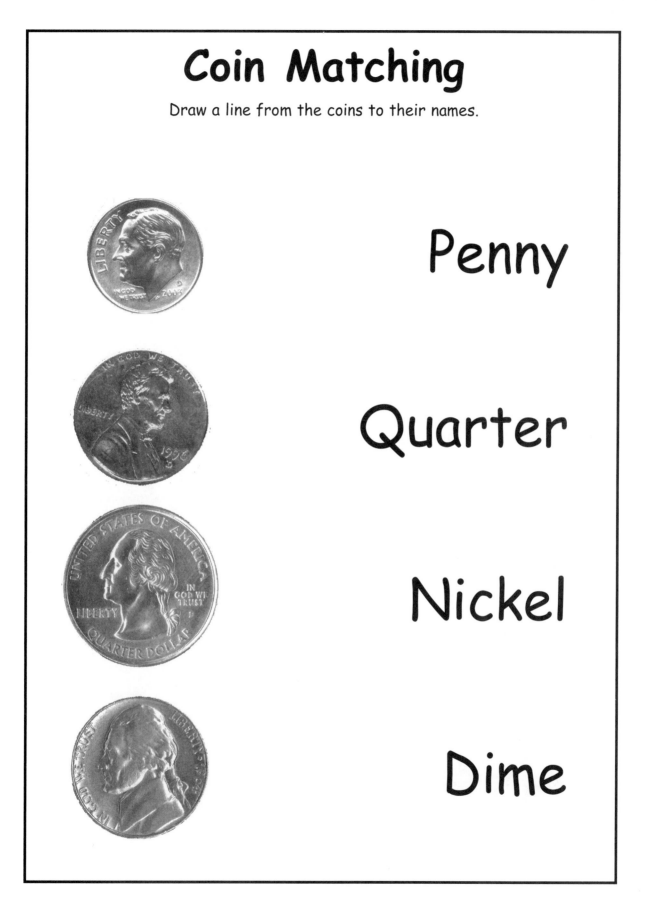

Penny

Quarter

Nickel

Dime

Coin Matching

Draw a line between the coins and their numbers.

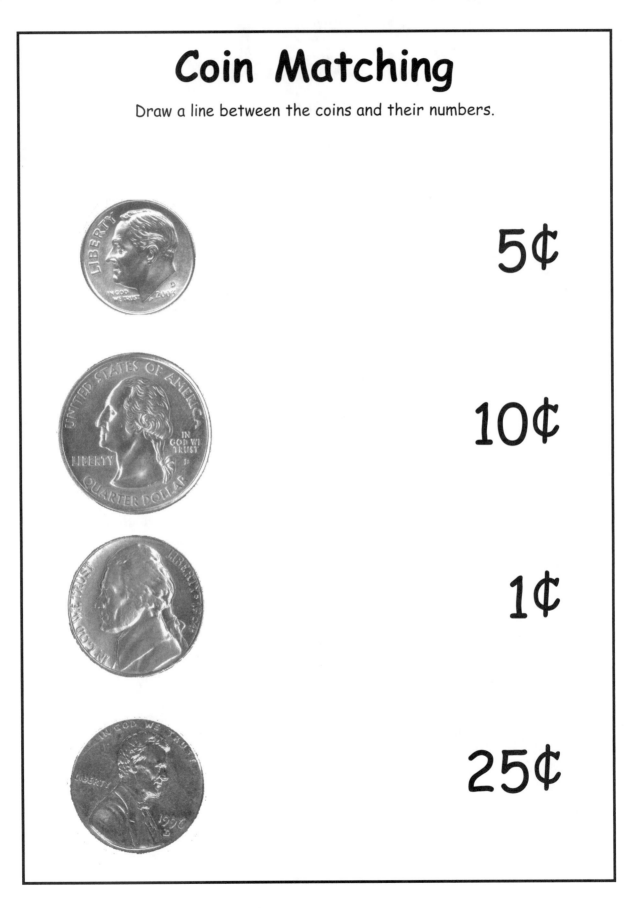

Paper Money Matching

Draw a line from each bill to the correct dollar amount.

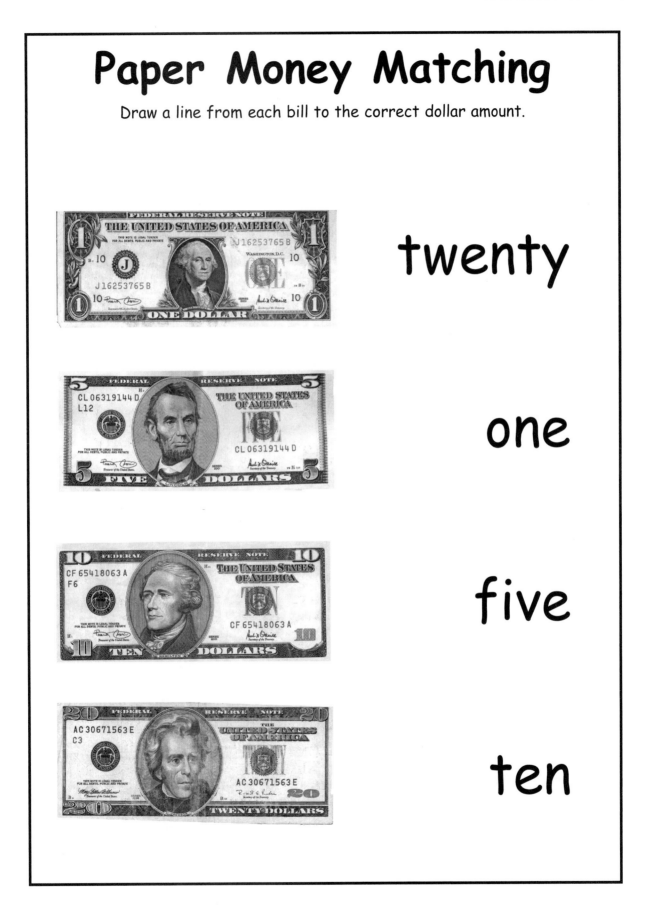

twenty

one

five

ten

Paper Money Matching

Draw a line from each bill to the correct dollar amount.

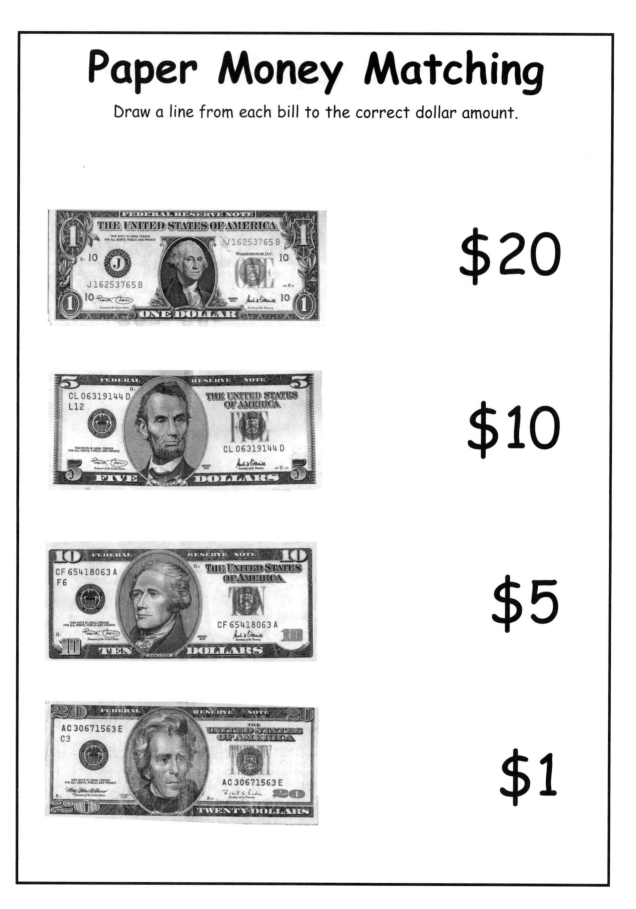

When you are out and about, or even at home, there are things you need to know to stay safe.

Know Your Signs

Color the lights green, yellow and red.

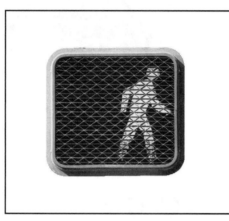

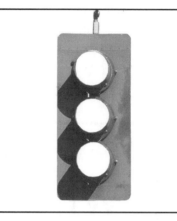

Color the bottom light green.

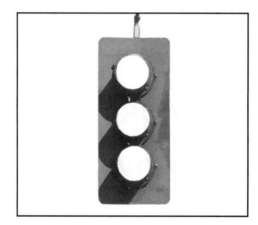

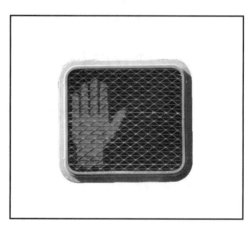

Color the middle light yellow.

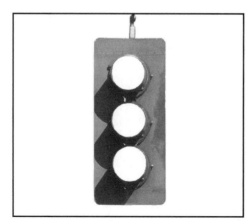

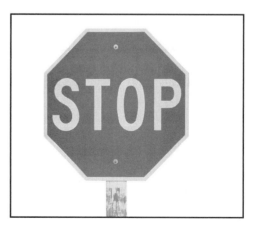

Color the top light red.

 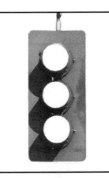 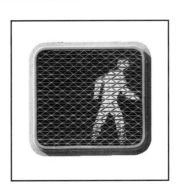

Color the bottom light green.

All these signs mean WALK.

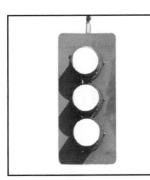

Color the middle
light yellow.

Yellow means the green

light is about to change to

red.

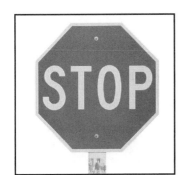 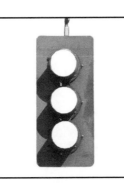 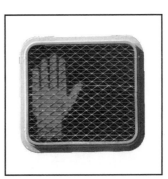

Color the top light red.

All these signs mean STOP, DON'T WALK.

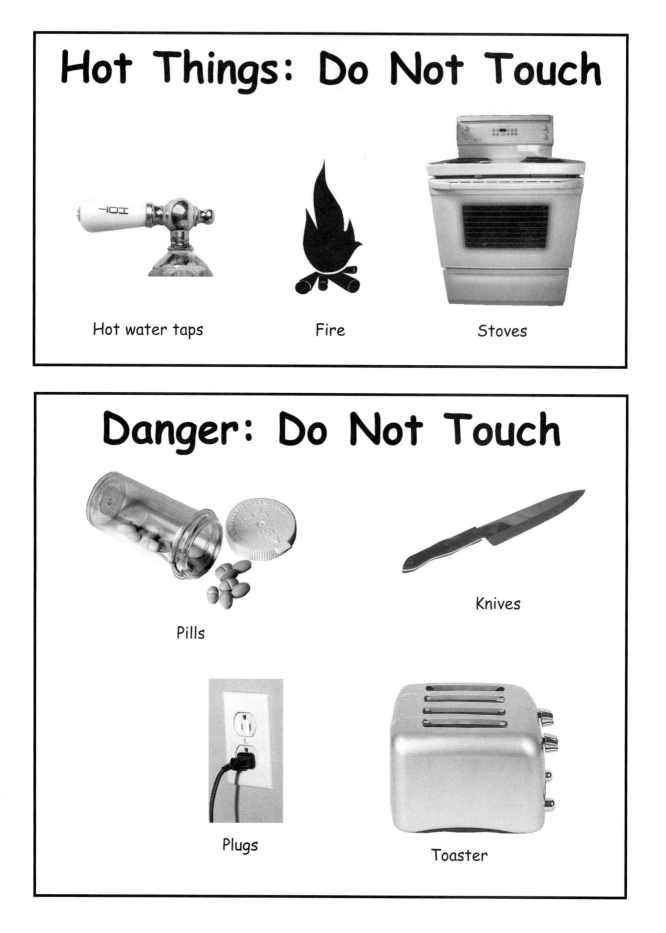

Hot Things: Do Not Touch

Hot water taps

Fire

Stoves

Danger: Do Not Touch

Pills

Knives

Plugs

Toaster

PART THREE

✢

Tear-outs

Choice Cards

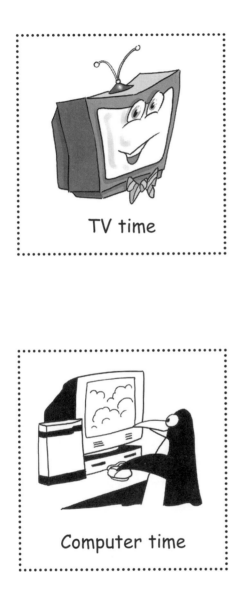

TV time

Computer time

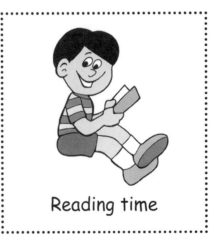

Reading time

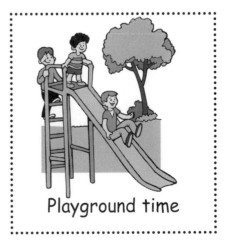

Playground time

Choice Cards

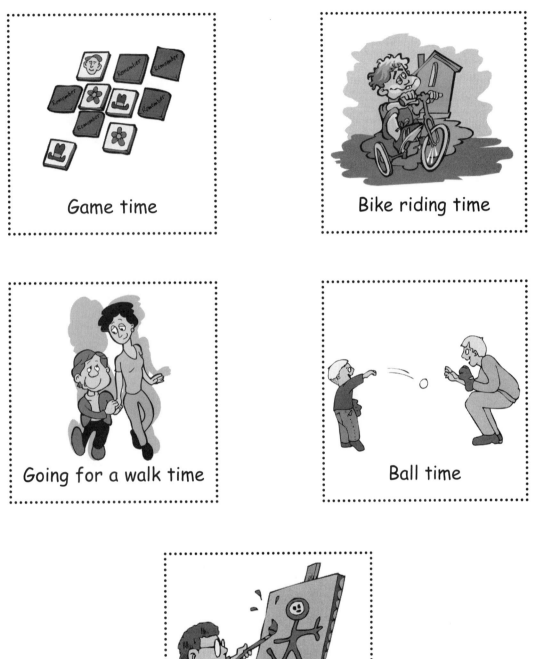

Game time

Bike riding time

Going for a walk time

Ball time

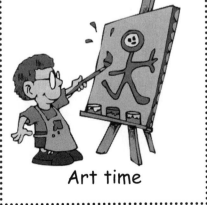

Art time

Sequences for Calendars

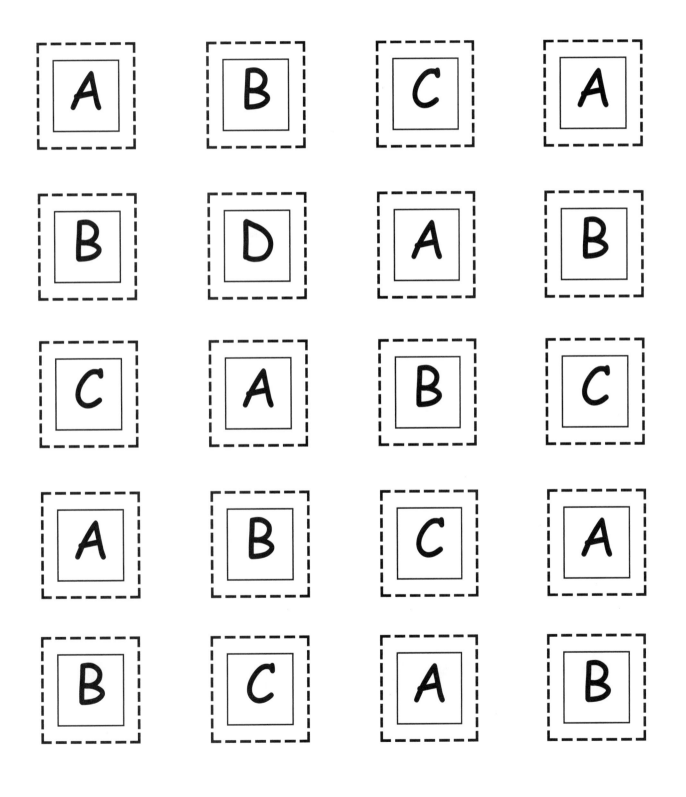

Sequences for Calendars

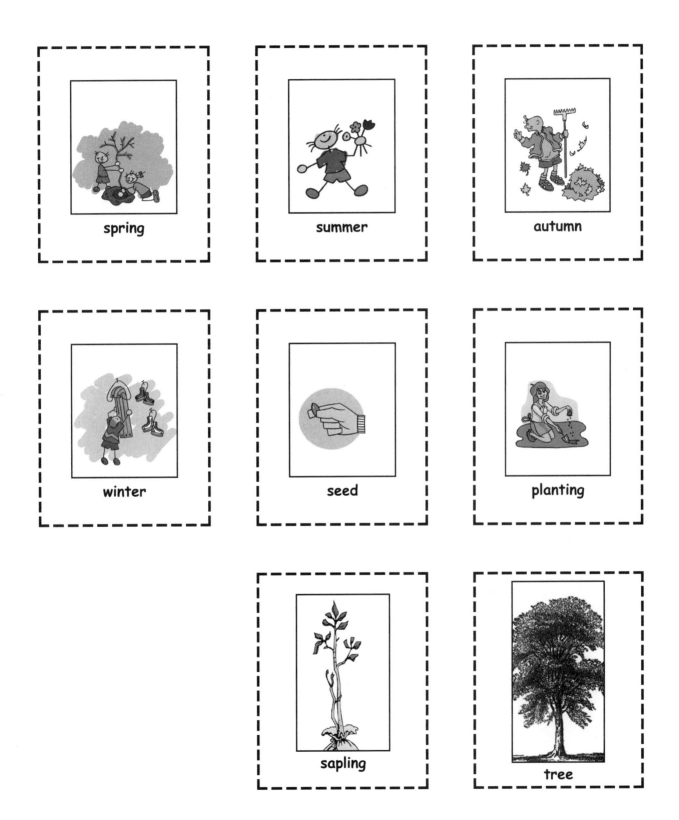

Sequences for Calendars

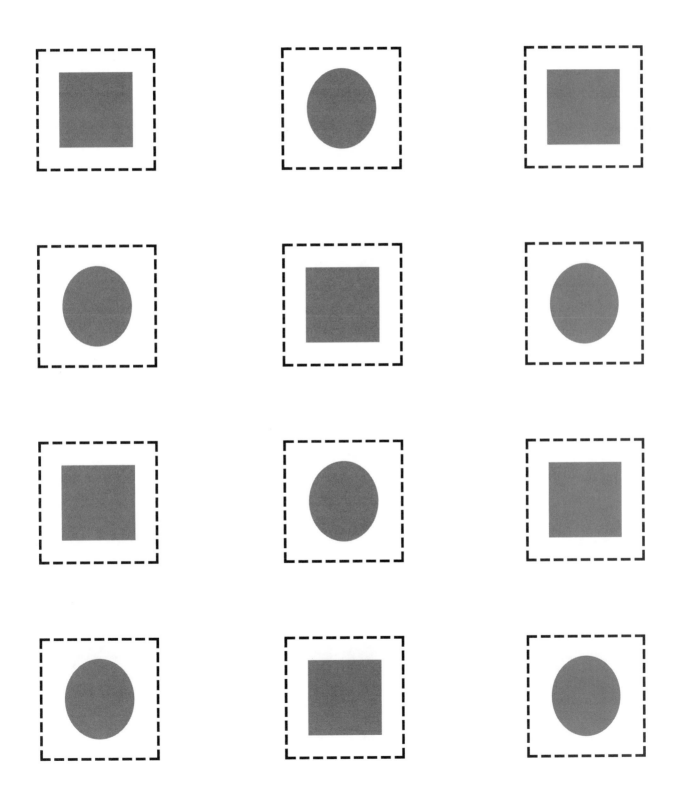

Sample Clock Face

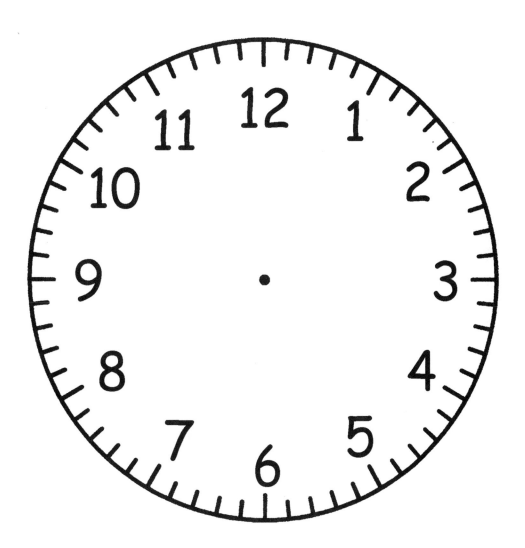

(We suggest you have this page laminated or placed into a plastic protector so that you can draw clock hands over and over with dry-erase markers. Alternatively, you can mount the page on cardboard and make clock hands out of a sturdy construction paper, held in place with a brad.)

"Don't Look at Me That Way" Cards

My child is on the
Autistic Spectrum.

For more information about autism
go to:
www.autism-society.org

My child is on the
Autistic Spectrum.

For more information about autism
go to:
www.autism-society.org

My child is on the
Autistic Spectrum.

For more information about autism
go to:
www.autism-society.org

My child is on the
Autistic Spectrum.

For more information about autism
go to:
www.autism-society.org

My child is on the
Autistic Spectrum.

For more information about autism
go to:
www.autism-society.org

My child is on the
Autistic Spectrum.

For more information about autism
go to:
www.autism-society.org

A Sample Letter
for Your Doctor or Dentist

Dear_____,

This is a letter of introduction. My child will soon be visiting your office. He is a special needs child on the autistic spectrum. As you may know, interactions with strangers are very stressful for such a child. I am trying to make this visit easy for all of us.

Is it possible for us to visit your office prior to the scheduled appointment so that my child can become familiar with the surroundings as well as with you and your staff? This may make the actual appointment more successful. I realize that you are very busy, and I will understand if this would not work out.

If you would like to know more about autism prior to this visit, I would be happy to send you pertinent information. You can also find information on the following website: www.autism-society.org.

My child has a difficult time expressing his feelings, and any supplementary knowledge you have may make it easier for you to communicate with him.

One aspect of life that is particularly difficult for children on the autistic spectrum is their lack of a concept of time. Having to wait in a waiting room is difficult for any child. It is even more so for mine. If possible, I would like to arrange for us to be your first appointment of the day. This will ensure there will be less disruption to your office.

If an anesthetic needs to be used, please note that it may excite my child, since children on the autistic spectrum often respond to sedatives in a contrary fashion.

Please share this letter with your office staff so that they will be prepared for our visit as well.

We look forward to meeting you.

Sincerely,

A Sample Letter for Your Hairdresser, Shoe Store Clerk or Anyone You Feel Is Appropriate

Dear_____,

    This is a letter of introduction. My child will be visiting your establishment soon. She is a special needs child on the autistic spectrum. As you may know, interactions with strangers are very stressful for such a child and I am trying to make this visit as easy as possible for all of us.

    If you would like to know more about autism prior to this visit, I would be most happy to send you pertinent information. You can also find information on the following website: www.autism-society.org.

    My child has a difficult time expressing her feelings, and any supplementary knowledge you have may make it easier for you to communicate with her.

    We look forward to meeting you.

Sincerely,

The Basics about Autism: What You Should Know

The following definition is from the Autism Society of America: Autism is a severely incapacitating lifelong developmental disability that typically appears during the first three years of life. It occurs in approximately fifteen out of every 10,000 births and is four times more common in boys than girls. It has been found throughout the world in families of all racial, ethnic and social backgrounds. No known factors in the psychological environment of a child have been shown to cause autism. The symptoms are caused by physical disorders of the brain. They include:

1. Disturbances in the rate of appearance of physical, social and language skills.
2. Abnormal responses to sensations. Any one or a combination of senses or responses are affected: sight, hearing, touch, pain, balance, smell, taste and the way a child holds his body.
3. Speech and language are absent or delayed, while specific thinking capabilities might be present.
4. Abnormal ways of relating to people, objects and events.

SIGNS OF AUTISM

- No pointing by one year
- No babbling by one year; no single words by 16 months; no two-word phrases by 24 months
- Loss of language skills at any time
- No pretend playing
- Little interest in making friends
- Extremely short attention span
- No response when called by name; indifference to others
- Little or no eye contact
- Repetitive body movement, such as hand flapping or rocking
- Intense tantrums
- Fixations on a single object, such as a spinning fan
- Unusually strong resistance to changes in routines
- Over-sensitivity to certain sounds, textures or smells

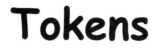

Tokens

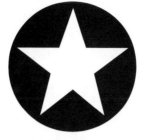

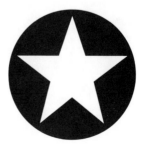

Other Ulysses Press Mind/Body Titles

The Autistic Spectrum:
A Parents' Guide to Understanding and Helping Your Child
Lorna Wing, M.D., $14.95

Uses the latest developments to improve communication, develop potential abilities and expand social interaction.

Smiling at Shadows:
A Mother's Journey Raising an Autistic Child
Junee Waites & Helen Swinbourne
Introduction by Lorna Wing, M.D., $14.95

An insightful and honest account of the often-difficult path to adulthood that a child "on the spectrum" must face. It is also the story of two parents who learned how to step into their child's world and draw him out into their own.

Know Your Body: The Atlas of Anatomy
2nd edition, Introduction by Emmet B. Keeffe, M.D., $14.95

Provides a comprehensive, full-color guide to the human body.

101 Simple Ways to Make Your Home
& Family Safe in a Toxic World
Beth Ann Petro Roybal, $9.95

Sheds light on common toxins found around the house and offers parents straightforward ways to protect themselves and their children.

How to Meditate: An Illustrated Guide
to Calming the Mind and Relaxing the Body
Paul Roland, $16.95

Offers a friendly, illustrated approach to calming the mind and raising consciousness through various techniques, including basic meditation, visualization, body scanning for tension, affirmations and mantras.

To order these books call 800-377-2542 or 510-601-8301, fax 510-601-8307, e-mail ulysses@ulyssespress.com, or write to Ulysses Press, P.O. Box 3440, Berkeley, CA 94703. All retail orders are shipped free of charge. California residents must include sales tax. Allow two to three weeks for delivery.

About the Authors

Phil Abrams is a father, husband, behaviorist, actor and now writer. A graduate of UC Berkeley, he is soon to receive his Masters in Special Education from National University in Los Angeles. Phil recently served as a technical advisor for autism on an episode of the "The District" and has also created a script about an autistic young man's journey—the way he perceives the world differently, and how that difference changes others' perceptions. It is his hope to see it brought to life on television.

Leslie Henriques, M.P.H., is the co-publisher of Ulysses Press and a graduate of UC Berkeley. She received her Masters of Public Health degree from the University of Hawaii, Manoa. Leslie lives in Berkeley, California with her husband, Ray Riegert, and two children, Alice and Keith. Her nephew Elijah Abrams has inspired her to publish books that empower parents of children with autism.

Lorna Wing, M.D., an internationally recognized medical authority, has been studying autism for over 30 years. She is also the mother of an autistic daughter. Her work with autistic children in the 1970s redefined the classic profile of autism and helped create the concept of autistic spectrum disorders. Throughout her career, Dr. Wing has developed practical and constructive ways for parents to cope with the wide range of difficulties experienced by families caring for autistic children. She is the psychiatric consultant for the National Autistic Society in the United Kingdom and her numerous books and papers have been translated into several languages. She lives in East Sussex, England.